God
And
Cancer

A DIY Healing Perspective

A God And Series Book

Edward G. Palmer

God *And* Cancer

God _And_ Cancer
A DIY Healing Perspective

Edward G. Palmer

God *And* Cancer: A DIY Healing Perspective

Publisher:

JVED Publishing
13570 Grove Drive #361
Maple Grove MN 55311
http://www.jvedpublishing.org

Paperback Edition
ISBN 9798323901319
All Rights Reserved

Disclaimer: This book is the sole opinion of the author based on his research, knowledge, and understanding. It is not intended to provide medical advice and is solely for educational purposes. Anyone in need of medical assistance should seek the appropriate expertise within the medical industry.

Scripture References: All references to Scriptures in this book are taken from the New King James Version (NKJV) unless otherwise indicated by a three to seven-character translation code as shown on pages 8-9.

Capitalization Protocol

On all Bible citations, regardless of the translation used and where the context clearly points to God ALMIGHTY or to Jesus Christ, this book distinguishes between the two. This is done by using either small-cap characters or lowercase characters.

For God Almighty, a small capitalized style protocol is followed and reflected in the format: CREATOR, FATHER, ALMIGHTY, GIVER, HE, HIS, HIM, HIMSELF, YOU, YOUR, ME, MINE, MOST HIGH, MY, MYSELF, LORD AND SAVIOR, ETC.

For Jesus Christ, a lowercase protocol is used except for Lord and Son. Hence, when these pronouns are used for Jesus, they show up as: he, his, him, himself, you, your, me, my, myself, savior, Lord, or Son.

This has generally been followed throughout the book but is not the case with every cited verse. It is used for those verses in which the context cannot be easily disputed, or in the case of citing, a quality or attribute which belongs solely to God.

For those interested in the original translation capitalization, the author refers them to the actual Bible version used for the cited text. A list of Bible translations is shown on the next page. In other cases, capital letters used within the mentioned sentence structure were also changed on common words for ease of reading or modern grammar. In other cases, the capitalized letters were left as shown in the original translation. Hence the original Bible phrase "; Because" might appear as "; because." In all instances, the author maintains complete integrity of translation, and the writings herein can be traced back to the original Bibles to confirm the accuracy of presentation. While not perfect, the capitalization protocol is reasonably consistent and enhances the reading and value of the author's writings.

Bible Translations

KJV	King James Bible [1]
NKJV	New King James Version [2]
AMP	Amplified Bible [3]
ASV	American Standard Version [4]
BSB	Berean Bible Study [5]
CEB	Common English Bible [6]
CEV	Contemporary English Version [7]
CJB	Complete Jewish Bible [8]
CSB	Christian Standard Bible [9]
DB	Darby Bible [10]
DRC1752	Douay-Rheims Challoner 1752 [11]
EMTV	English Majority Text Bible [12]
ENO	Book of Enoch - Laurence 1883 [13]
ESV	English Standard Version 2016 [14]
GNB; GNT	Good News Bible or GNT *Translation* [15]
GNBA	Good News Bible with Apocrypha [16]
GNV	Geneva Bible 1560 [17]
GW	God's Word Bible [18]
HCSB	Holman Christian Standard Bible [19]
HEB	Hebrew Bible - JPS 1917 Edition [20]
ISV	International Standard Version [21]
JSB	Jewish Study Bible [22] - 1985, 1999
LIV	Living Bible [23]
MACE NT	Daniel Mace's New Testament 1729 [24]
MEV	Modern English Version [25]
MLT	Morris Literal Translation [26]

MOFF	James Moffatt Translation [27]
MSG	The Message Bible [28]
NAB	New American Catholic Bible [29]
NABRE	New American Bible - Revised Edition [30]
NASB	New American Standard Bible [31]
NASB77	New American Standard Bible 1977 [32]
NASB1995	New American Standard Bible 1995 [33]
NASB2020	New American Standard Bible - 2020 [34]
NCV	New Century Bible [35]
NET	New English Translation [36]
NET1	New English Translation - First Edition [37]
NIV	New International Bible [38]
NIV2011	New International Bible -2011 Edition [39]
NJB	New Jerusalem Bible [40]
NLT	New Living Translation [41]
NMV	New Messianic Version Bible [42]
NRSV	New Revised Standard Bible [43]
NRSV-CI	NRSV - Catholic Interconfessional [44]
NRSVUE	New Revised Standard Bible - 2021 [45]
REB	Revised English Bible [46]
RSV	Revised Standard Version [47]
SET	Simple English Translation [48]
TAN	Jewish Tanach - Stone Edition 1996 [49]
TEV	Today's English Version [50]
WEB	Webster's Bible [51]
WEY	Weymouth's NT [52]
WESLEY NT	John Wesley's New Testament [53]
YLT	Young's Literal Translation [54]

*Dedicated to everyone who takes responsibility
for their own health and healing!*

Table Of Contents

Part I

DIY Healing Your Spirit

1 Introduction   17

2 Cancer Strikes   23

3 The Understanding Heart   29

4 The Stress Solution   39

5 When The Soul Leaves   51

6 The Appointed Time, Part 1   63

7 The Appointed Time, Part 2   69

8 The Appointed Time, Part 3   83

9 Jesus Always Healed?   105

10 Death Cheated   117

Part II

DIY Healing Your Body

11 Water & Healing   129

12 Cancer 101   149

13 Nutrition & Cancer   155

14 Sugar & Cancer   169

15 Food & Cancer   171

16 Exercise & Cancer 177

17 Teeth & Cancer 185

18 Sleep & Cancer 193

19 Microbiome & Cancer 201

20 Cancer Healing Protocols 205

21 Cancer Resources 231

Back Matter

Notes 244

Bible Translation Notes 260

About The Author 267

Author & Publisher 268

Related Self-Care Health Books 269

Other Books & Writings 271

A Real Salvation Prayer 272

A special thanks to my wife Becky for her creative thoughts, editorial inputs, and encouragement.

PART ONE

DIY Healing Your Spirit

CHAPTER ONE
Introduction

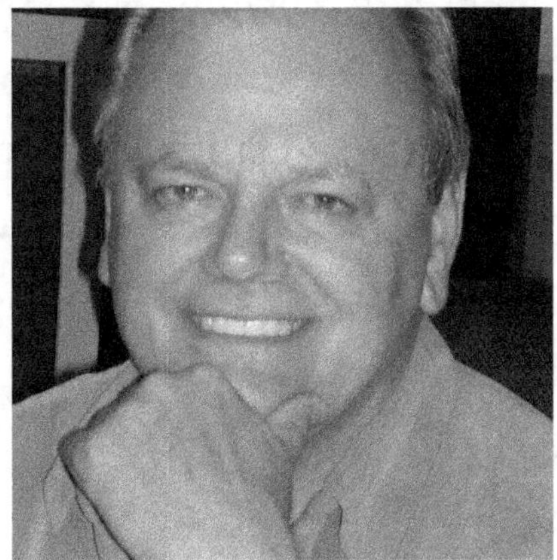

Edward G. Palmer

Hello, and thank you for reading this book: "**God _And_ Cancer:** *A DIY Healing Perspective.*" I am author Edward G. Palmer. For 50 years, I have practiced "Healing Self-Care[1]." Any vocation or calling practiced for 50 years will make you somewhat of an expert in that area of study. Therefore, it's common for people to seek out my thoughts on Healing Self-Care.

A   detailed   author's   website   is   at   http://

www.edwardgpalmer.com. You will find a complete bio and other information there, including my health and healing blog. On this site, you will find other books on health and healing. Having lost my first wife to pancreatic cancer after 39 years of marriage and being a spiritual man, I wrote a small book about what the Bible says about healing[2]. I now have over 50 years of experience with alternative healing strategies.

I wrote the second health and healing book while I was recovering from a stroke. It left me seeing double and severely impaired my eyesight at age 76, but I am healed.

I explained the approach to my healing in this book and how family, friends, and doctors became severely concerned when I refused to get an MRI to check for brain tumors. You'll find a detailed DIY[3] approach to alternative health and healing in this book - *"The Doctor's Death Diagnosis[4]."* You will also find a list of *"100 Healing Secrets & Tips"* that is not widely known, not even by health professionals.

My third health and healing book, published in late 2023, is *"Healing Self-Care Primer: How To Create a DIY Self-Care Health & Healing Program[5].* This book teaches you how to create a self-care healing program that helps you avoid drugs, doctors, and hospitals. See notes for further information.

These health and healing books and my website blog

on health and healing constitute my effort to help people understand they have many low-cost options for healing other than going to the doctor or hospital. I write about cost-effective alternative health and healing strategies. Once you accept responsibility for your health, there is a DIY way to care for your health and healing. You don't have to become financially drained or bankrupted by an expensive and out-of-control allopathic medical insurance industry.

Is It Health Care - Or A
Health Protection Racket?

That is the first question in the *Healing Self-Care Primer* book. What is your opinion? Has healthcare become out of control and too expensive for many people and families in the United States? Is there a need for more DIY self-care instructions so that people can relearn how to take care of their medical issues?

Are Cancer Cures Suppressed?

I was ordained in 2000 and have written several books on Christianity. This book is dedicated to all of those who have struggled or died from cancer. I lost several family members to cancer. Most recently, I lost a niece to a particularly aggressive form of cancer. Before that, I lost my first wife, and before that, her father died of colon cancer. A cancer diagnosis can be a death sentence, but it doesn't have to be one.

In June 2003, I lost my first wife[6] to pancreatic cancer. Everything seemed well except for an irritating gas bubble along the left side of her body, about even with her waist. Her pancreatic enzymes were tested, but they were all in the normal range.

The doctors then went down through her throat to check out her stomach, and everything was normal. The next test involved a CAT scan. That is when the doctors found a tumor on her pancreas that engulfed her spleen. Spots were also seen on her liver, indicating the cancer had metastasized onto her liver and spread perhaps to some other parts of her body.

The last test was invasive, and the surgeon went down and took a sample of the tumor. It was indeed pancreatic cancer, and it was stage IV, having spread to other parts of her body. The doctor informed us she had as little as 10 days to live and perhaps several weeks and maybe even a few months if she was lucky.

My first wife lasted 98 days before she died of pancreatic cancer and got her heavenly wings. Before she died, I spent weeks digesting cancer information and seeking a cure. At this writing, I've now spent months of my life digesting hundreds if not thousands of pages of cancer information. To my amazement, I have found many alternative cures for cancer that are being hidden by the traditional allopathic medical industry. There are simple cures, such as eating the seeds in apples, apricots, and other fruit seeds, which can also prevent you from getting cancer in the first place. Why is this information about additional cancer cures being hidden?

All I learned came too late to save the woman I loved for 43 years. Having traveled in charismatic churches, many Christians believe that healing doesn't occur because a person's faith is not strong enough. I have even heard some preachers preach that if you are sick, it is because you are living in sin. Such teaching is not of God.

There are two primary questions I will answer in this book.

Will God heal everyone who prays a prayer of faith, or is that Christian mythology? Secondly, what can you do for yourself if you actually have cancer? The answers might surprise you.

In later chapters, you will find protocols for fighting cancer from an alternative nutrition or nutraceutical approach. Finally, I have a Bonus website page where I post additional information on how to cure cancer. Check here[7] for the latest information or DIY, easy-to-use cancer resources I feel are essential for you to know.

It is my prayer that *God <u>And</u> Cancer* will become a valuable healing resource for you and your family in your own or your family's struggle against the ravages of cancer.

May God heal you or your loved one from the disease of cancer. If HE chooses not to, may you and your loved one find HIS peace that indeed does pass all human understanding. That is a gift HE gave my beloved first wife.

CHAPTER TWO
Cancer Strikes

-- My First Wife's Last 98 Days On Earth --

"But those who seek the LORD shall not lack any good thing." Psalm 34:10

"But if they refuse to listen to [God], they will perish ... and [they will] die from [a] lack of understanding." Job 36:12 NLT

"He [or she] shall die for lack of instruction." Proverbs 5:23

"MY people are destroyed for lack of knowledge." Hosea 4:6

"I will be gracious to whom I will be gracious, and I will have compassion on whom I will have compassion." Exodus 33:19

"I will have mercy on whom I will have mercy."
Romans 9:15

David said: "Who can tell whether the LORD will be gracious to me, that [my] child may [be healed]? But now [that] he is dead; why should I fast? Can I bring [my son] back again? I shall go to him, but he shall not return to me." 2 Samuel 12:21-23

Jesus said: "Nor can they die anymore, for they are equal to the angels and are sons [and daughters] of God, being sons [and daughters] of the resurrection." Luke 20:36

Jesus said: "When I sent you without money bag, knapsack, and sandals, did you lack anything?" So they said, "Nothing." Luke 22:35

This book contains spiritual advice for those who stand with God's Word. These people have consciously chosen to walk in God's light and now realize they are destined for HIS eternal life. Some secular people and some who identify as Christians may object to some discussions in part or in whole. However, I aim to teach God's people what HIS Word says about divine healing.

Will God always heal people because of their or others' healing prayers? The short answer is No!

Prayer: May God's grace, peace, and mercy be with you this day and always. Edward

In 2005, I procrastinated on writing this information. I knew I would suffer some emotional stress to write what God wanted me to write here. Just counting the days my first wife lived after February 26, 2003, brought some tears. That was the worst day of my life. It was the day that she and I were told of her inoperable pancreatic cancer.

It wasn't the worst day because of that diagnosis. Listen, I believe in divine healing, and I had already prayed for her through two separate times when she was coughing up blood clots from her lungs. Both of those events were life-threatening and scary. No, this was the worst day of my life because God had confirmed to me, as HE had told her, that her remaining time on earth was now very short.

While dying, she looked at me sadly and said: "My job on earth is done, and it is time for me to go home." Thinking about those words coming from her mouth can easily make me tear up. That is because emotions are stored with our memories in the recesses of our brains.

You can relive an event if you dig deep enough in the mind. Looking into her eyes, I knew that her time on earth was nearly over, as God confirmed the same to my spirit. There would not be another miraculous healing in her life. The doctor said she might have as little as 10 days.

If we were lucky, she might have a few months. Stunned, we drove silently back to our home in Elk River from the Hennepin County Medical Center in Minneapolis, where she had the internal ultrasound and biopsy test.

That night, I found myself gasping for air, as I couldn't breathe. I also couldn't sleep, and the pain in my chest was overwhelming. The pressure on my chest was heavy, and it felt like an Elephant was sitting on top of my chest. I didn't know if my body could breathe without my wife beside me. For that matter, I didn't know if I really cared. For the moment, thoughts of checking out myself flowed freely. I knew I was ready to go home to be with God. I had been prepared for a life after this earthly one for twenty-five years.

Now, I wondered if I could even live without her. Indeed, my worst fear in this earthly life had now manifested itself. God had set my wife and me on a path of physical separation. It was a path that would return me to my own flesh, a path that no longer would include my wife and me as one flesh. As events progressed, I could feel the cords that held our flesh together as one begin to separate. She was being prepared for a heavenly journey. I was being prepared for a life without her. I knew she would be fine. Myself? There were a lot of tears and lonely thoughts at that moment. We both had our lives flash before us and cried a lot together. I began to think about what could be done.

The big question is: "Will God always heal as a result of prayer?" I've already given you a short answer. I will explain the basis for that answer from God's Word. I will use my first wife's life, cancer, and death to illustrate for you what God wants you to know about healing.

CHAPTER THREE
The Understanding Heart

Let's discuss the Christian belief system and what Jesus said in Matthew 13:15 about understanding with our hearts. This is related to the spiritual and metaphysical issues of healing.

Jesus said: "For the hearts of this people have grown dull. Their ears are hard of hearing, and their eyes they have closed, lest they should see with their eyes and hear with their ears, *lest they should understand with their hearts and turn [to God's righteousness],* <u>*so that I should heal them*</u>**." Matthew 13:15**

Jesus is teaching us that if we could only understand with our hearts and turn to God's righteousness -- he would be able to heal us. For this to happen, we must open our eyes and see and open our ears and hear what he is teaching.

He may be speaking to Christians in the 21st Century.

For the most part, Christianity is in error and believes that Jesus is God. It is part of the religion's false Trinity doctrine. Suppose you want to know why Trinitarianism is a false doctrine. In that case, the answers are in my book, *"God And Jesus: The Identity Crisis."*[1] However, for our illustration here, consider the following three simple statements of Jesus. Nobody needs a theological degree to understand these teachings of Jesus. You only have to accept what Jesus teaches as the gospel truth.

Jesus said, "But now you seek to kill me, a Man *who has told you the truth which I heard from God."* **John 8:40**[2]

Jesus answered them, saying, "Who is my mother, or my brothers?" And he looked around in a circle at those who sat about him, and said, "Here are my mother and my brothers! *For whoever does the will of God is my brother and my sister and mother."* **Mark 3:33-35**

Jesus said to her, "Do not cling to me, for I have not yet ascended to my FATHER; but go to my brethren and say to them, 'I am ascending to *my FATHER and your FATHER, and to my God and your God.'* **" John 20:17**

Jesus teaches us that **he is a man**. He also has family

relationships and teaches that **he is a brother** to everyone who does the work of his FATHER. For me, that means Jesus is my brother, not my God. What about you? Jesus goes on to tell us that his God is ours. That his FATHER is our FATHER. It means Jesus has a God that he worshipped; he was a human male and is a brother to every person who truly believes in what he taught in the New Testament. In other Scripture, Jesus teaches us to worship his FATHER. How did Christians evolve to ignore the teachings of the savior they claim for eternal life?

The entire dogma of the Trinity doctrine is complicated, so I wrote a book on the subject. There are many theological points to discuss and examine closely. That is especially true regarding theological doctrines like the "I AM" (Greek ego eimi) self-identifying statements in the Gospel of John. Scholars ignore a blind man who used the exact words.

From my perspective, Christians have been subjected to gaslighting for over 2,000 years. Furthermore, the Orthodox Church actively teaches against what Jesus taught in the New Testament. I've attended Catholic, Lutheran, Presbyterian, Church of Christ, Assemblies of God, and Charismatic Churches like the Association Of Faith Church Ministries (AFCM). Eventually, I spent four years in a Christian cult, observing for God what was taking place. Aside from the gaslighting about who God really is with the Trinity, I observed thieves and crooks occupying Christianity's pulpits.

That has led me to believe that the Trinity doctrine has led many believers to think their evil behavior and sins are covered by the blood of Jesus. See Hebrews 10:26, which no doubt was written to dispel this false idea for people whose behavior was similar in ancient days.

Could belief in the Trinity preclude people who identify as Christian from getting into Heaven? The answer is **Yes** -- **IF** that trinity belief leads them to conclude that they can freely sin in this earthly life and / or if they worship Jesus instead of God.

The answer is **No** -- **IF** that trinity belief does not involve their unrighteousness[3], willful sin, and idolatry. In other words, they worship Jesus' God, not Jesus[4].

In the first case, the unrighteous Christian is firmly condemned to Hell for their belief that sin is now somehow okay through Jesus Christ. They have literally treated the blood of Jesus Christ as a common thing and insulted God's Spirit of grace. This is equivalent to crucifying Christ on the cross again. Study Hebrews 10:26 if this is unclear to you. Continued sin should be a "fearful thing" for all believers. Even worse are those who engage in idolatry, worshipping Jesus. See Revelation 2:4 for the discussion of our FIRST Love[5].

In the second case, the righteous (Trinity-believing)

Christian is just another example of a child of God who is confused about Jesus's identity. They are no different from a Jewish, Muslim, or other child of God who also does not understand Jesus. Remember, "Practicing righteousness[6] makes us righteous just like Jesus Christ."

"Children, do not be misled: anyone who does what is right is righteous, just as Christ is righteous." 1 John 3:7 REB

When you walk in God's light as Jesus Christ did, you have escaped the pollution of this world. There is no going back. It is a one-way street.

"People can know our Lord and savior Jesus Christ and escape the world's filth. But if they get involved in this filth again and give in to it, they are worse off than they were before." 2 Peter 2:20 GW

I want to mention all of this to make something clear. Accepting Jesus Christ in your heart should be a new beginning for you with God. It is a time to grasp God's hand and let HIM guide you. It should not be the end of some spiritual quest. Some churches put people through a confirmation process. They accept Christ and become a church member at the end of that process.

The next duty is usually to make a pledge of money to the church. Often, this is the last time the person picks up a Bible. Such a church has failed God. Instead of teaching the beginning of a new life with God, some confirmation classes teach young people that they have learned all they need to know about God. When you accept Christ as your savior, you begin a new walk with God for the rest of your life. That is salvation!

Christ Is A New Beginning,
Not The End Of A Journey!

I have been told several times that I am fearless. Indeed, I stopped fearing man some time ago. However, I do sincerely fear my God. What is often mistaken as fearlessness is simply a strong confidence in God.

"In the fear of the LORD there is strong confidence, and HIS children will have a place of refuge." Proverbs 14:26

When you reach this level of confidence in God, it won't matter what your checkbook looks like or how the world treats you. It also won't matter if your truck gets a dented driver's side door because you hit someone's bumper. Nor will it matter if you think you are unlucky and others get all the breaks in life. Strong confidence in God is what you get when you walk in His light.

I tell you this because earlier, when I wrote this text, I only had exactly $76.62 to my name. Yes, it can cause some stress if you let it. That afternoon, my daughter also informed me that she had dented the passenger's door on her husband's new Chevrolet truck. Yes, that, too, can cause some stress if you let it. However, if you walk in God's light, you have to look upward and not around you from an earthly perspective.

Decades ago, a friend taught me that you need to **pray it up** to God and **play it down** on this earth during times of trouble Those are good spiritual words of advice. As long as you focus on God, you will have perfect peace. This is what Isaiah has taught us. Take it to heart and see what God will do for you.

"God will keep you in perfect peace, when your mind is stayed on HIM, because you placed your trust in God." Isaiah 26:3 [Ed's Paraphrase]

When you seek God, you can understand why the Psalmist teaches that you will not lack any good thing in Psalm 34:10. You will also understand why Jesus asked the question to his apostles: "Did you lack anything?" The answer was no, even when Jesus sent them out without money. I have lived through a cycle of almost zero cash with God many times. I am a witness to the fact that God has always made a way where there seemed to be no way. Admittedly, such times will test your faith in God.

Despite my strong confidence in the LORD and HIS ability to take me through yet another cash flow crunch, I have learned something about this physical realm. I have learned that even though I think I am doing well, my body might inform me that I am not doing well. To the degree we can walk with our spirit, all is well. But, if the flesh gets some control, stress will manifest in our bodies. This is true whether or not we will admit it or, for that matter, whether we even realize it.

Do you listen to your body? I can absorb an incredible amount of stress. I will still be standing when all around me are totally stressed out. Why I am like this, I do not fully understand. I have a natural desire to trust in God and operate in faith. This is not to say that stress doesn't rack my body at times, as it does. I have also experienced a mind-body separation. This happens when you think you are well, but your body tells you something different.

Therefore, low stress is an attribute of healing. My first wife and I were under enormous stress the three years before her cancer death. There is little doubt that it impacted her more than I, even if she hid it somewhat. In the realm of cancer invading our bodies, stress is one of the major contributing factors.

Your peace in this earthly life will be directly proportional to your ability to yield your life over to God's control. It is not easy and not necessarily related to whether one is saved or has obtained eternal salvation. It's strong faith. See the following graphic illustration.

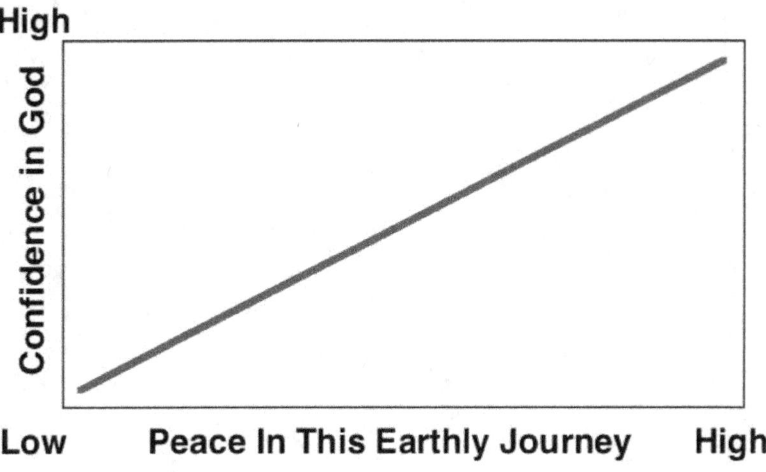

Strive for a stress-free life. That statement might seem like a fantasy, but achieving a significant degree of peace is possible. Trusting in Jesus' teachings will give you high confidence in his God. If you can "understand with your heart," it can open a pathway for Jesus to heal you.

CHAPTER FOUR
The Stress Solution

The preceding graph shows that your peace in this earthly journey will be proportional to your confidence in God. High confidence in God brings you perfect peace. Low confidence in God will bring anxiety and uncertainty. No matter where you think you are with your spirit and mind, the body you possess may have different thoughts. I wish I could tell you that I continually operate as I do now, where I have a perfect peace knowing that God is in control; I can't.

At times, I, too, suffer. The difference for me is that I know that to the degree I do suffer a lack of peace, it is because I am not in God's presence. I return to prayer and worship when I become aware of a lack of peace. It is my spiritual cue that I am "in the world" and not "in His peace." It is a time to mentally refocus on God and get out of myself or this world.

If life is getting you down, maybe it's because you are too focused on yourself or the things in this world. Pick up a Holy Bible and start to read. Shift your thoughts towards God. If you do not know where to begin in the Bible, start at Psalm 34. This Psalm is an excellent place to meditate when you are hurting and in trouble. Listen to a part of this Psalm of David.

"The righteous cry out, and the LORD hears, and delivers them out of all their troubles. The LORD is near to those who have a broken heart, and saves such as have a contrite spirit. Many are the afflictions of the righteous, but the LORD delivers him [or her] out of them all." Psalm 34:17-19

Norman Vincent Peale taught me that problems constitute a sign of life. When confronted by a congregation member complaining of his many issues, Norman asked him if he would like to move to a place where 100,000 people lived, and no one had a problem. The man answered yes, he would like that.

Norman replied: "Okay, but it's Woodlawn Cemetery in the Bronx, and everyone is dead." Norman concluded that it then seemed logical that problems constituted a sign of life. If you walk with God in righteousness and HIS light, "Many will be your afflictions." That is what God's Word teaches. Why? It is simple. Satan doesn't care if you are "into yourself" or "into this world." He only cares about those who are "into righteousness" and belong to God.

Do not be concerned about your afflictions if you are righteous. God will be near your broken heart, comfort you, and deliver you out of your troubles. You should be concerned when life is peaceful, you have no trouble, and everything seems to go your way. As Norman Vincent Peale taught: "Without some problems in your life, you might be on your way out." Or, at the least, you are of no concern to Satan. Lack of trouble in this earthly life could be a sign you are living on the wrong side of the fence, which is called righteousness. That reality might signify that you are of the world, not God's light. Check your priorities.

God Will Comfort Your Broken Heart!

When I used to think that my wife would not be available to share life anymore, I experienced a broken heart and unimaginable sadness. I cannot live with those kinds of thoughts because to do so is to live in the past with all the continued pain of her death. I can only live in the present moment. She is not a part of my life anymore, and I must move on in life and put her death behind me. I can take comfort from God knowing that she is now with HIM. When the sad thoughts arrive, I replace them with good thoughts, memories of our life together, and the blessing that I know she was to me.

"Blessed be the God and FATHER of our Lord Jesus Christ, the FATHER of mercies and God of all comfort, who comforts us in all our tribulation, that we may be able to comfort those who are in any trouble, with the comfort with which we ourselves are comforted by God." 2 Cor. 1:3-4

Regarding healing in our bodies, we must move beyond our problems and allow God to deal with them. Many times in my life, I have not been able to understand something. During those times, I can choose certain anxiety or let go and give the issue to God. My solution is what Norman Vincent Peale taught: put the issue(s) or problem(s) into a gunnysack labeled--"I can't handle it, LORD!"

How To Empty The Gunnysack

You may have already mentally collected many such objects and need help figuring out what to do with them. I can also imagine that you carry the objects in a gunnysack over your shoulder, and they are now a heavy burden on your life. You may even have become quite irritable about these issues or problems. Maybe you feel unlucky, and everything seems to happen only to you. You might even be frustrated and angry at those who love you. If this sounds like you, you have a high-stress level and must unwind a little. Norman taught me another lesson that I adopted over four decades ago. It has never failed me once over the years.

Imagine that all your troubles, irritations, and afflictions are in that sack on your back in the form of pots and pans. Each pot and pan represents a troubling issue that increases your stress in this earthly life. Each item means something over your head that you can't understand, make sense of, or worry about. Now imagine that Jesus Christ is standing before you and asking you to take on his yoke so you can rest. Christ is trying to tell you there is more to life than you can realize with your human senses.

In that moment, Christ also asks that you give him all your pots and pans, everything that burdens and troubles you in this earthly life. You take one item at a time out of your gunnysack and give it to Christ. Eventually, your gunnysack becomes empty, and all the troubles of your life are now taken off your back. You are not free of issues or problems. However, you now have heavenly help from God and His Son Jesus.

Jesus said: "Take my yoke upon you and learn from me, for I am gentle and lowly in heart, and you will find rest[1] for your souls." Matthew 11:29

"Give all your worries and cares to God, for HE cares about what happens to you." 1 Peter 5:7 NLT

"When troubles come ... sing HIS praises [from within your heart] with much joy." Psalm 27:5-6 LIV

"My brethren, count it all joy when you fall into various trials." James 1:2

Those Who Endure This Earthly Life Are Counted As Blessed!

"Indeed we count them blessed who endure [life]. You have heard of the perseverance of Job and seen the end intended by the LORD -- that the LORD is very compassionate and merciful." James 5:11

If you want healing in your own life or more peace, a good place to start is to lower the level of stress you are experiencing. One of the greatest joys of my life occurred during my wife's illness. It was watching her settle into the loving arms of God. I watched her transcend all the cares of this world and only look forward to the joy of her heavenly home. The transformation that took place before my eyes brought both joy and tears. I felt joy from watching her experience the perfect peace of God's presence. Indeed, the whole family experienced God's presence in our home and is a witness to her perfect peace. The tears came from just knowing that her earthly life was nearing its end.

Reflecting on what I witnessed can quickly grab my throat and cause more tears. Yet I know that these could be tears of joy or sadness. I spent 43 years loving this woman, and in this earthly life, I could never give her the peace that God brought her during the last 98 days of her life.

Verily, I say to you that at any moment in your earthly existence, the level of peace you can experience will range from virtually none to virtually perfect peace. The choice will be yours to make.

My wife had struggled to understand how to get to that area of perfect peace, but in the end, God gave it to her during the last 98 days of her life. To the degree you can have high confidence in God, you can shed your earthly concerns. It comes from a heart that totally surrenders itself into God's hands. My wife was like Martha in Luke 10:41. She was a servant of God but was always concerned about hospitality issues. I.E., Making sure everyone was fed, etc. She was a quintessential caregiver to my children, grandchildren, family, and friends. However, in the end, she was able to give herself entirely over to God and let HIM take over all of her concerns. Only then could she empty her gunnysack.

The peace my wife exhibited while dying was only matched by her unbelievable bravery. I do not recall her ever expressing a concern about herself. I only remember her expressing concerns about others. The 98 days God gave us allowed everyone to say our goodbyes. In the end, there was no fear in her -- only peace! I praise the God I serve for the incredible gift of total peace that HE gave my wife before she passed.

Of course, our individual faith plays a role in healing, and I am always conscious that the prayers of a righteous man count a lot with our God. I remember looking at my wife's somewhat emaciated body towards the end, wondering how our grandson Christopher was coping. He was our first grandson and spent his first 24 months with us. It established a soul bond with my wife as if he was her son. At age 15, he fought back the tears and kept praying. I remember thinking towards the end what an excellent healing story it would be to see her suddenly get up, having experienced yet another miracle.

I could almost read Christopher's mind as he thought the same thing I did: "It's not over yet. God still has time to heal her." It wasn't over yet, and who knew whether God would be gracious in this situation? To paraphrase King David, "Who knows what God will do now?"

I have lived a high-tension entrepreneurial life and studied stress reduction more than once. My top three methods of dealing with stress are simple. It starts with my spiritual connection to God. I assume you've taken time to empty your gunnysack and are not holding onto emotions or traumas mentally which are beyond your ability to control.

Three Ways To Reduce Stress

1. Prayer
2. Nutrition
3. Exercise

Draw near to God[2] and witness that HE will draw near to you. Give God 100% of your heart, and you will see miracles. It doesn't always mean your prayers will be answered exactly how you want them answered. Indeed, my prayer for healing my first wife's cancer was not. Yet I understand that all of this was God's will, even if I did not understand what would happen next in my life. I knew that my wife's death was something that must be placed into the "I can't handle it, LORD" gunnysack.

For me, God will have to deal with every aspect of her death and absence from my side. I will get my chance to understand when I join her in Heaven. God has said: "Do not lean[3] on your own understanding." Make God integral to your life; you'll find HIS peace.

Stress takes over life just like pain takes over life. When your body is in pain, all of your body's resources are working to deal with the pain. I am happy my wife was relatively pain-free except for two bad days. This in itself is unusual for pancreatic cancer, which can be pretty horrific. A variety of pain medications were used to keep her pain-free so her body could do its best with its God-given innate healing powers. She was conscious until the last 24 hours of her life when it became necessary to dramatically increase her pain medications. Did her pancreas burst open or start to leak? The chemicals inside the pancreas cannot exist outside of it except within the intestinal area. It is like an acid that would literally eat through all of the other organs.

About four hours before my wife took her last breath, our dog Annie jumped up on the bed beside her and howled aloud. She immediately left the bed and never came back. It was the first time our cocker spaniel ever howled, and it left all of us wondering at the time what it was all about. She was almost nine years old and was my wife's dog. By spiritual reckoning, we believe my wife's soul left her body then. The event that her dog Annie signaled was the departure of her spirit soul. It took about four more hours before her body stopped breathing on its own.

CHAPTER FIVE
When The Soul Leaves

Suppose you can understand that my wife's spirit soul actually left her body before her body physically stopped functioning in all respects [stopped breathing, heart stopped, etc.]. In that case, you can understand why Jesus told the thief next to him that he would be in Paradise that day with Jesus.

The soul doesn't need transportation to Heaven, nor does it wait for all bodily functions to cease. When the soul leaves the body, it takes off for home. We knew that my wife's essence [her spirit soul] was nowhere to be found in the bedroom by the time her body ended its last physical function. It was self-evident she had gone home. The fact we observed this spiritual reality gives credence to a statement in the Gospel of Phillip about Jesus' physical death.

From the Gnostic Gospel of Philip, we read the following:

"Those who say that the Lord died first and then rose up are in error, for he rose up first and then died. If one does not first attain the resurrection will he not die? As God lives, he would already be dead." ...

"While we are in this world, it is fitting for us to acquire the resurrection for ourselves so that when we strip off the flesh, we may be found in rest." ...

"Those who say they will die first and then rise are in error. If they do not first receive the resurrection while they live, when they die they will receive nothing."

Suppose you can understand why her spirit soul rose before her body died. In that case, you will also understand these words of Jesus Christ concerning our entering into life at the point of the spirit soul leaving our body. It should be sufficient enough for you to understand that our resurrection will occur at death. The new resurrection body, like Christ's, will be a gift at a later appointed time.

Jesus said: "If your hand or foot causes you to sin, cut it off and cast it from you. It is better for you to enter into life lame or maimed, rather than having two hands or two feet, to be cast into the everlasting fire.

And if your eye causes you to sin, pluck it out and cast it from you. It is better for you to enter into life with one eye, rather than having two eyes, to be cast into Hell fire." Matthew 18:8-9

Christ makes it abundantly clear that we enter eternal life when we die. The Gospel of Philip clarifies that you better get your [eternal] "life" here while on Earth because you won't get it after you leave [the Earth]. So, the essence of life is what lies inside us. Our bodies are like the gloves worn on our hands during cold weather. When a hand is inside the glove, the glove becomes animated and appears alive. Take the hand [our spirit soul] out of the glove [our body], and the glove [our body] becomes lifeless.

Philip's Gospel further clarifies the separation of our spirit soul from our physical body with the following statement about Jesus Christ.

"My God, my God, why, O LORD, have you forsaken me?" To which Philip teaches us: "It was on the cross that [Jesus] said these words, for it was there [on the cross that] he was divided."

Note: Philip teaches us that Christ's spirit soul was "divided" and separated from his body [and rose] before the death of his physical body. Christ's separation of the spirit soul from his body is an example of what we can expect at the time of our death. The resurrected body was given to Christ later, just like ours will be given to us at a later [appointed] time.

It was sometime in the mid-1960s that my first wife and I were asked by her Uncle Earl to go to the hospital and help make a decision as to whether or not he should pull the life support from his wife, her Aunt Bernice, who had been in an accident. This was in San Diego, California, when I was in the Navy. It was our first experience with life support machines, and we were young adults. I can still remember the hospital room and Aunt Bernice lying in the bed with a mechanical respirator. She could not breathe for herself, and she had no brain activity. Her heartbeat was strong.

I remember that I could clearly see that Bernice exhibited no essence or life force. It was because Aunt Bernice's spirit soul had left to go home. It only took a few minutes to agree to turn off the respirator that kept her lungs working. Aunt Bernice stopped breathing a few moments after the respirator was shut down. Her heart stopped beating shortly after that. I knew, at that time, it was the right decision.

Nothing has changed in over fifty years that would alter that decision. Aunt Bernice, like my first wife, had left her earthly body and just wasn't there even though we could artificially keep her body going. I can imagine that just as my wife took her last two breaths, we could have attached a respirator to her body to keep it artificially breathing, but why? She wasn't there. To keep her body parts functioning just because we couldn't cope with her "shedding her flesh" would have been ungodly.

Today, medical science has advanced far ahead of where it was in the 1960s. Suppose you place a feeding tube directly into the stomach of an almost dead body and combine it with IV fluids, antibiotics, medications, and oxygen machines. In that case, you could keep a human body going almost indefinitely. This is very true if there exists no pathological disease eating away at the human body, such as pancreatic cancer.

We even have machines to keep the heart going, shocking it back into operating condition or forcing it to contract and expand with electrical signals as needed. In essence, all that is left to do is to keep moving the body periodically to prevent skin ulcers from forming.

After our experience with Aunt Bernice, my wife and I agreed that neither would want machines to keep our bodies going over a protracted period. It is a hideous and even evil thing that people do when they cannot let go of a loved one whose spirit has left the body or is unduly entrapped in a body that can no longer function with a mind as God designed.

When Do You Remove Body Support Machines & Nutrition?

The controversy over keeping a human body going indefinitely was center stage in the societal debate over whether or not to remove the feeding tube from Terri Schiavo in Florida. The discussion was likened to starving her to death by "refusing" to give her food. However, if God wanted us fed with a stomach tube supplied externally with food, HE would have equipped our bodies with such a tube and provided attendants 24 hours a day to meet our needs.

Suppose the idea of dehydration during the death process seems repulsive to you. In that case, you are ignorant of the body's natural dying process. Naturally, the spirit rejects food and nutrition as it shuts down the body in the dying process. In fact, food can cause more pain in the body as the spirit soul attempts to shut things down and exit this Earth, shedding its human flesh. Medical interventions can unduly restrain a spirit soul from leaving Earth.

Do you believe it is righteous to keep someone on a feeding tube indefinitely? For fifteen years? It is unrighteous and self-serving to those who cannot cope with death. It is also shameful to state that it is wrong in the eyes of God to remove a feeding tube kept in for so long.

This isn't a right-to-life issue like abortion, which kills a fully functioning human. This is about the right to die a natural death with some amount of dignity after a long period of exhaustive medical intervention in the mechanically untethered body that God Almighty gave us. Terri died on March 31, 2005, 13 days after her tube was removed for a third time.

If you think it was wrong in God's eyes to remove Terri's feeding tube, I want you to show me a single case in the Bible where it took God fifteen years to heal someone. That is how long Terri's body was kept alive by family intervention. God doesn't need hours, days, weeks, months, and years to heal anyone. Every case of healing in the Bible was instantaneous in nature. Yet Terri's body was kept artificially alive for fifteen years by medical intervention.

A body like hers could be kept going for another 40 years if no pathological disease attacks it. Terri lived a God-given natural life for 26 years. Then, people who claim to love her refused to let her die a God-given natural death after eight years of exhaustive medical intervention and seven years of subsequent litigation. Some people even wanted to keep her mindless, brain-damaged body artificially alive indefinitely using medical technology.

Is that love? No, it is sick, perverse, and cruel. It is the action of spiritually ignorant people who lack true faith in God. After her feeding tube was removed on March 18, 2005, Congress passed a law to save her by authorizing Federal Court intervention. At one point, Florida's Governor even considered a plan to have state agents seize her and reinsert the feeding tube. All the political efforts failed. Can you rejoice for Terri's new life? Jesus asked his disciples this question. Yes, there is emotional pain and trauma when a loved one dies. Yet Jesus says, "If we loved them, we should rejoice."

Jesus said, "You have heard me say to you, 'I am going away and coming back to you.' If you loved me, you would rejoice because I said, 'I am going to the FATHER,' for my FATHER is greater than I." John 14:28

The second time Terri's feeding tube was removed, Florida passed a law forcing it to be reinserted; it was declared unconstitutional. There is no reason to involve the government or court in a family's end-of-life decision. They will only prolong the family's grieving process. Many organizations & people have used Terri Schiavo for political purposes; God will repay!

Only the godly love of all family members can release an entrapped spirit soul and let its artificially fed body die. Was Terri inside her body after 15 years [of being brain dead]? Some say yes, and some say no. Did it matter? If she was still inside her body, her family and society long ago lost any spiritual perspective about a natural death for her. They unduly entrapped her spirit soul on this Earth in a body that lacked a cognitive mind, a body artificially kept alive.

In the other case, she was long gone and probably wondered why stopping the artificial means of keeping her Earthly shell and pseudo-life alive took so long. Yes, much controversy surrounded the participants in Terri's real-life and death drama. However, there was really only one central truth in the drama. Terri Schiavo's body was kept artificially alive by means that the Creator never intended to be used over a protracted period.

Without medical intervention, Terri would have died a natural death 7-15 years earlier in 1-2 weeks. There is a natural [nonintervention] death process of spirits shedding their flesh.

Here is some startling medical truth. Suppose you have good insurance and you are unlucky enough to get a feeding tube placed in your comatose or vegetative state body. In that case, you will likely remain that way until the medical insurance coverage ends, the family's money runs out, or the state refuses to pay for additional care. This is especially true when a caregiver or a loved one thinks they are applying a standard of true love.

Verily, I say to you that true love can place a comatose or vegetative state loved one in the hands of God after reasonable medical care has been exhausted. If you choose artificial means for keeping their body alive, you do so for yourself, not for them. It would be different if they were cognitive and gave those medical instructions, but it wouldn't be your decision.

Many people with quadriplegia have lived a meaningful life as a result of their own cognitive choices; Christopher Reeves is one example. However, it is their own spirit soul that is directing their physically impaired life choices. God certainly may have a role in helping them make meaningful decisions.

"Let love be without hypocrisy. Abhor what is evil. Cling to what is good." Romans 12:9

Take a deep breath and put yourself into the body of your comatose or vegetative state loved one. Ask yourself how long it would be reasonable if you were in that state. What would godly love do? If you think that love would be "long-suffering" in such an instance, you are misinterpreting the Bible. Keeping someone artificially alive is simply cruel.

It didn't take my wife and me long to realize we needed to put her Aunt Bernice into God's loving hands. The condition was beyond our understanding and the medical system's ability to cure. Bernice's life belonged in the category of "I can't handle it, LORD." Putting her into God's hands with prayer lets HIM decide about healing, life, and death. It is no more complicated than yielding to God what is beyond us.

Finally, my nephew was found in this unconscious condition. I went to the hospital several nights and prayed for him. The condition was beyond our understanding and the medical system's ability to cure. However, his eyes occasionally moved, and we could observe other autonomic physical activities. These movements came from his brain stem and were involuntary, even if they seemed synced to our conversation and touch. They were part of the body's autonomic nervous system. It doesn't mean conscious activity was present, but it can seem that way for some people. After a few days, the family had to let him go because, like Terri Schiavo, there was no brain activity, and my nephew had already left his body.

**The soul leaves the body,
Before the body itself dies!**

CHAPTER SIX
The Appointed Time, Part 1

Sudden Unexpected Deaths

When the Living Will became available in Minnesota, I completed one. I gave a copy to the local clinic I used. In that Living Will, I said it was okay to use machines on me for seven days if I could not speak for myself. After seven days, I asked that the machines be taken off of my body and that I be left in the arms of the Loving God that I trust. Should God desire me to stay on this Earth, I know that HE can perform the healing that my body needs. Should it be my time to go, I am more than ready. When you know your God, you know there is genuinely an appointed time to die. There is no need to fear an Earthly death by keeping your body artificially alive.

"And as it is appointed for men [or women] to die once, but after this the judgment." Hebrews 9:27

Note: We see in Strong's Concordance2 that the word

"appointed," as used in Hebrews 9:27, comes from the Greek word apokeimai (ap-ok'-i-mahee), which means to be reserved; fig. To await --be appointed, (be) laid up.

The word "appointed" means what it says. God has an appointed time for every one of us to die a natural death. This is when our spirit soul sheds off its flesh and goes home. We can keep God's appointed time when our bodies are not subjected to artificial life support over a protracted period. That is man's way of trying to cheat death, but it never works. However, it does feed bank accounts.

As I was initially writing this text many years earlier, news of the sudden death of the 11-year-old son of a friend of my family reached me. The boy was struck dead by a car while returning from the mailbox outside of his rural home, only a few miles from my home. It is nothing short of a Greek tragedy when any young person dies, especially a child. Hear my prayer, LORD!

Prayer: FATHER God, YOU see the immense pain we suffer when sudden death strikes any family member. As YOU have comforted me, I pray for those suffering from sudden death in the family that YOU would comfort them as in death, there is no absolute comfort other than YOURS.

FATHER, I also pray for the families of everyone whose

body is being kept alive by artificial means to delay their death or loss. Guide these families to make the right spiritual decisions for their loved ones so that these spirit souls may not be trapped needlessly on this earthly plane by a love that fails to acknowledge the eternal rest that awaits all righteous souls. Indeed, YOU are in control of these life-and-death matters. Indeed, both situations fit into the human gunnysack we all carry that says: "I can't handle it, LORD!"

Who can know our appointed time except God? When our oldest daughter Paula was 12 years old, my wife's cousin lost their 12-year-old son in a cruel motorcycle accident. It was one of the saddest funerals I have ever attended. It didn't take long for my wife and I to project this onto our daughter Paula, who was the same age. Isn't that what our human brains automatically do? "My God, what if that would have been our child?" Life has a way of offering up many things to think about when it comes to healing and death. Verily, I tell you that you will never know if today is your last day. Only God knows the times of our life and death during our Earthly journey.

Often, riches get our egos going, and we think we can escape the misery of living by buying our way out of life's troubles. This is one reason people are kept artificially alive for so long. They've got the money. When my wife became ill, our options were limited because our funds were non-existent. We chose to trust in God and do the best with what we had available. I shudder to think of what I might have put my wife through to save her had I been a multimillionaire with unlimited resources. That is the main problem with wealth. Man will trust in wealth before he trusts in God.

Jesus clarified that trusting in our wealth to live life or relying upon our resources instead of God's doesn't work. Here's an example.

"But God said to him, 'Fool! This night your soul will be required of you; then whose will those things be which you have provided?' " Luke 12:20

When it comes to death, no amount of money and medical technology we can muster will be able to alter God's decision even if we can keep a body artificially alive. What we can do is choose the direction we are going. For the 11-year-old boy who was suddenly killed, there is only one place you will find him. It will be in God's loving hands, who understands his short life. A few more years would have required that he make a conscious spiritual choice. Without making a spiritual choice at the time of our maturity (usually around 12-13), our behavior will demonstrate which side of life we chose, the world's or God's.

I attended the funeral of Connie's 11-year-old son. I can tell you that he had already chosen God. He touched many other lives in his short life and was loved by many; the funeral home was packed. Yet, can we say that the death of this young boy was at God's appointed time? It is hard because many other factors can affect or determine the length of our days.

The Power Of Prayer In Healing

King Hezekiah's story demonstrates that we do not know God's plan or timing for our death. It also indicates that sincere prayer from a dedicated and loyal heart can result in healing from God.

"In those days Hezekiah was sick and near death. And Isaiah the prophet, the son of Amoz, went to him and said to him, 'Thus says the LORD: Set your house in order, for you shall die, and not live.' Then he turned his face toward the wall, and prayed to the LORD, saying, 'Remember now, O LORD, I pray, how I have walked before YOU in truth and with a loyal heart, and have done what was good in YOUR sight.' And Hezekiah wept bitterly. And it happened, before Isaiah had gone out into the middle court, that the word of the

LORD came to him, saying, 'Return and tell Hezekiah the leader of MY people, Thus says the LORD, the God of David your father: I have heard your prayer, I have seen your tears; surely I will heal you. On the third day you shall go up to the house of the LORD. And I will add to your days fifteen years.' " 2 Kings 20:1-6

Because of Hezekiah's sincere prayer, God healed him and extended his life on this earthly plane by fifteen years. That is the power of a righteous individual's prayer.

CHAPTER SEVEN
The Appointed Time, Part 2

32 Issues Affecting Healing

I believe the following thirty-two issues are involved with cancer, healing, and death. The list may be incomplete, but I know these healing attributes must be considered. These items help us understand what our human body is facing on Earth. Some items have already been discussed. My plan is to discuss all of them.

1. Stress
2. Pain
3. Our Faith
4. Other's Faith
5. Our Prayer
6. Other's Prayer
7. God's Sovereignty
8. God's Grace
9. God's Mercy
10. God's Healing

11. God's Glory
12. God's Bigger Picture
13. God's Protection
14. Good Habits
15. Bad Habits
16. Sin
17. Repentance
18. Age or Youth
19. Lack of Faith
20. Lack of Knowledge
21. Nutrition
22. Body's Innate Healing Ability
23. Health Laws
24. Food Laws
25. Sanitation
26. Doctors
27. Traditional Medicine
28. Alternative Medicine
29. Anointing With Oil
30. Call To Elders
31. Pray For Yourself While Healthy
32. God's Call to Pray for Someone Else

I believe that all of the items listed above affect cancer, healing, and death. God's Word speaks directly to most of these items. The above list is neither prioritized nor all-inclusive. You can see that prayer is only a part of a longer list of items that will affect our bodily healing.

If You Love Me

I remember a time when I would have told you that if I am sick, do not bring anyone to me that would pray a prayer with the words to "heal me if it is THY will, LORD." This was biblical ignorance for me at that time.

At the time, I was one of those Charismatic folks who would have been insulted if you even suggested that God might not want to heal my sickness or disease. Why, for Heaven's sake, man [woman], don't you know the Word of God? Yes, I would have uttered those words. I was programmed with mythology instead of God's Word. Instead, I would say: "Bring me people who will pray knowing that it is God's will for me to be healed." Perhaps you are one of my Charismatic or Pentecostal brothers or sisters who currently hold that opinion? Well, guess what? If you have that opinion, it does not represent the truth of God's Word for you, and you should keep reading.

I have altered my thinking due to the understanding given to me by God. Today, I would have people pray for my healing if it were God's will. Sometimes, it is not HIS will for healing if healing means a longer life on Earth. It might be that the healing God wants for us is to take us to our heavenly mansion and give us rest from this earthly life and its incumbent struggles.

That is what God did for my wife. In God's bigger picture, it was her appointed time to go home. Her healing was the gift of eternal rest for her soul in a heavenly mansion God prepared. Can you understand that such a transition and shedding of the flesh is also a blessing? If not, why? The death of my wife was not the answer I sought with my prayers, yet it was still a great blessing to her from God. I had come to spiritual maturity and could condition my prayers to God with the words: "THY will be done, O LORD!"

Jesus said: "If you loved me, you would rejoice because I said, 'I am going to the FATHER.' " John 14:28

Do you rejoice when a loved one goes to the FATHER? Jesus clarifies that you would rejoice if you knew he was going to the FATHER and loved him. Perfect peace, perfect joy, and rest. We have long ago lost the ability to rejoice when a righteous person sheds their flesh to return to the FATHER. Yet rejoicing is what we should do.

How Much Grieving?

I know that some family members might think I didn't grieve enough over the loss of my wife. However, exactly how much should I grieve when God's Word tells me to rejoice? The answer might surprise you and is also in God's Word. You'll find instructions on grieving in the book of Sirach, Chapter 38.

"My child, let your tears fall for the dead, and as one in great pain, begin the lament. Lay out the body with due ceremony, and do not neglect the burial. Let your weeping be bitter and your wailing fervent; make your mourning worthy of the departed, for one day or two, to avoid criticism; then be comforted for your grief.

For grief may result in death, and a sorrowful heart saps one's strength. When a person is taken away, sorrow is over, but the life of the poor weighs down the heart. Do not give your heart to grief; drive it away, and remember your own end.

Do not forget, there is no coming back; you do the dead no good, and you injure yourself. Remember his fate, for yours is like it; yesterday it was his, and today it is yours.

When the dead is at rest, let his remembrance rest too, and be comforted for him when his spirit has departed." Sirach 38:16-23 NRSV

Be Comforted For Them
When Their Spirit Departs!

We should rejoice and be comforted at the death of our loved ones when we know they are in the hands of our God. I can tell you that I suffered many years over the loss of my first wife. Even so, life gives no respite from further heartache. Connie's son's death was also close to my heart. She was almost like another daughter, having been raised with my kids in the neighborhood and having known her for thirty years. To see her and her family suffer in such pain was almost unbearable.

Yet I eventually could "let my wife's remembrance rest," as Sirach teaches. What does Sirach mean? He means that I should stop constantly thinking about her daily. It means that I put my first wife out of my mind. That happened when anyone close to me died. After a period of grieving, I realized that I had to move on mentally. God and time will heal our broken hearts; I know!

Sirach also contains essential instructions on using the help of medical doctors and pharmacists. Listen to Sirach.

"Honor physicians for their services, for the LORD, created them; for their gift of healing comes from the

MOST HIGH, and they are rewarded by the king. The skill of physicians makes them distinguished, and in the presence of the great they are admired.

The LORD created medicines out of the Earth, and the sensible will not despise them. Was not water made sweet with a tree in order that its power might be known?

And HE gave skill to human beings that HE might be glorified in [their] marvelous works. By them the physician heals and takes away pain; the pharmacist makes a mixture from them. God's works will never be finished, and from HIM, health spreads over all the Earth." Sirach 38:1-8 NRSV

You can clearly observe that we should recognize medical resources regarding our illnesses. Nor are we to treat our bodies poorly. Many people today violate biblical health and food laws by eating or drinking items their bodies were not designed to consume. There are many excellent books written about biblical nutrition. Get some to read and start observing what you are doing to your own body.

If you smoke and drink alcohol, you are slowly poisoning your body. This has led many to a premature death. Instead of the natural death God had planned, many shorten their lives with poor health habits. When asked if smoking would keep someone out of Heaven, a pastor I know answered, "No!" He added, "It will help get you to Heaven faster!" When you treat your body poorly, you sin against your own body and accelerate your own earthly "shedding of the flesh."

"Or do you not know that your body is the temple of the Holy Spirit who is in you, whom you have from God, and you are not your own?" 1 Cor. 6:19

If you are a sharp reader, you might deduce that such sins against the body are both willful and continuous within many people. You might ask: "So will these willful sins now keep us out of Heaven?" This is a good question; the answer is also in the Bible. Consider these verses.

"Parents must not be put to death for the sins of their children, nor the children for the sins of their parents. Those worthy of death must be executed for their own crimes [sins worthy of death]." Deut. 24:16 NLT

"If anyone sees a fellow-Christian committing a sin which is not a deadly sin, he should intercede for him, and God will grant him life--that is, to those who are

not guilty of deadly sin. There is such a thing as deadly sin, and I do not suggest that he [or she] should pray about that. Although all wrongdoing is sin, not all sin is deadly sin." 1 John 5:16-17 REB

Apostle John clarifies that we can intercede with God for others when their sin is not a "deadly sin." Further, John says that God will grant them "life" when we intercede for them. I guess the idea that all sin is the same in God's eyes is really the stuff of Christian mythology. Obviously, there are some nuances with God. Rahab the harlot's lie to protect the Israelites is another example of nuance with God regarding sin. One of the cases where we can intercede with prayer for a loved one is when someone is hurting their body by a bad health habit.

My first wife and I started smoking when we were young. In our youth, we were told smoking was good for us. I managed to quit early. She struggled with cigarettes until the end, albeit she had slowed way down to about 6-7 cigarettes a day for years. In the last few weeks, she smoked 1-3 cigarettes a day. Her smoker's cough stopped years ago when she slowed dramatically down and even quit smoking completely for a while.

A few years before her death, she encountered a health problem, and she suddenly started coughing up blood clots about the size of a nickel. To say we were both horrified is an understatement. As she went through various medical tests, I kept interceding for divine healing. I prayed for each test to come back negative, and they did.

I believe my prayer for my wife fits the framework of Apostle John's teaching. My wife was healed, and we never found out what was wrong. I rejoiced because I knew the power of God healed her. About 2-3 years later, another bout occurred, which was even worse. The blood clots were more extensive this time, about the size of a quarter.

Again, I went into prayer mode, and she was healed. My wife then underwent very sophisticated medical tests, and they all returned negative. The final one was to go down into her lungs with a scope and look. I prayed that God would make her lungs look like she had never smoked in her life. A smoker's lungs look really black compared to the pinkish tissue of a nonsmoker's lung.

I was in the room as the doctor went down into her lungs with an optical scope to inspect her lung tissue. I remember how befuddled he looked as all he could see was normal, healthy lung tissue. I specifically asked him: "What did you see?" He told me that he only saw healthy lung tissue and did not find anything. Again, my wife was healed, and the doctor surmised that she probably had a tear on the lung tissue that was responsible for the blood. The doctor never really found anything solid. I knew that, once again, God healed her.

How did I pray? I got close to God in my spirit. I envisioned that God's hands were going over every area of my wife's body and organs that needed to be healed. As I saw HIS hands touching her organs and body, I saw HIS healing over those areas that needed a healing touch. I have used the same method to pray for several other healings. I also meditated and spoke God's Word about healing from a list I have written in my Bible.

Back To The Tumor Test

Back in the hospital on February 26th, while awaiting my wife's test results, I was reading healing verses and studying the Bible. **I kept focused on Luke 8:50. Jesus says: "Do not be afraid; only believe, and she will be made well."** As I waited for my wife to return from her invasive tests, I kept praising God and saying -- "I believe FATHER!"

This time, there would not be a divine healing. Like Apostle Paul, my prayers ran up against God's grace. And like Paul, God's grace would have to be sufficient, for I did not have any answers that made sense to my limited human understanding. My wife's sickness would have to be stuffed into the "I can't handle it, LORD" gunnysack this time. We never stopped praying for her healing right up to the end. We also never stopped praising God for the gift of my wife's life.

Smoking is a contributing factor in cancer, and so is any form of alcohol. My wife liked to have a Bacardi rum and diet-coke drink. She was a social drinker who finally stopped drinking before her last Christmas. Over 75% of pancreatic problems are associated with alcohol. It usually results in pancreatitis, a severe illness in which the pancreas stops functioning to some extent. Smokers also have a 2-4 times higher risk of developing pancreatic cancer than nonsmokers.

In some of my wife's last words, she wrote: "Could I have caused the cancer? Maybe! But not on purpose." Not one of us knows. My wife led a pretty healthy and clean life overall. She was also a very healthy eater. It could be that her pancreatic cancer could have been prevented if we had just planted her garden the year before.

Her pancreas was tested early on, and all its functions were within standard zones. Go figure. It can all boil down to a lack of nutrients at the cellular level within my wife's body.

Bad Life Habits Vs. Deadly Sins

We can contrast our typical bad habits and the sins against the temple of our body [overeating, obesity, smoking, moderate drinking, purging, lack of exercise, etc.] with what the Apostle Paul refers to as the "works of the flesh" in Galatians 5:19-20.

Paul teaches us that those who practice the works of the flesh "will not inherit the kingdom of God." Here is Paul's list of seventeen items we should be concerned with regarding eternal life. One can observe that the world is filled with people who live daily with these works of the flesh. Some Christian ministries even teach that a few of these flesh works are okay with God. Note that the list does not reflect what we would generally think of as bad health habits.

17 Sins That Can Lead To Spiritual Death

1. Adultery
2. Fornication (unmarried intercourse)
3. Licentiousness (sexual immorality)
4. Uncleanness
5. Idolatry
6. Sorcery
7. Hatred
8. Contentions

9. Jealousies
10. Outbursts of wrath
11. Selfish ambitions
12. Dissensions
13. Heresies
14. Envy
15. Murders
16. Drunkenness
17. Revelries Etc. (the like)

Don't Let Bad Habits Evolve Into Sin That Leads To Death!

CHAPTER EIGHT
The Appointed Time, Part 3

Thirty-Two Healing Verses[1]
For Your Prayers!

Note: All Verses From NKJV[2]

Exodus 15:26

"If you diligently heed the voice of the LORD your God and do what is right in HIS sight, give ear to HIS commandments and keep all HIS statutes, I will put none of the diseases on you which I have brought on the Egyptians. **For I am the LORD who heals you**."

Exodus 23:25-26

"So you shall serve the LORD your God, and HE will bless your bread and your water. And [HE][3] will take sickness away from the midst of you. No one shall suffer miscarriage or be barren in your land; [HE] will fulfill the number of your days."

Deuteronomy 7:15

"And the LORD will take away from you all sickness, and will afflict you with none of the terrible diseases of Egypt which you have known, but will lay them on all those who hate you."

Deuteronomy 32:39

"Now see that I, even I, am HE, and there is no God besides ME; I kill and I make alive; I wound and I heal; Nor is there any [one else] who can deliver [someone] from MY hand."

Psalms 6:2

"Have mercy on me, O LORD, for I am weak; O LORD, heal me, for my bones are troubled."

Psalms 30:2

"O LORD my God, I cried out to YOU, and YOU healed me."

Psalms 34:17

"The eyes of the LORD are on the righteous, And HIS ears are open to their cry."

Psalms 41:2-3

"The LORD will preserve him and keep him alive, and he

will be blessed on the earth; YOU will not deliver him to the will of his enemies. The LORD will strengthen him on his bed of illness; YOU will sustain him on his sickbed."

Psalms 103:2-3

"Bless the LORD, O my soul, and forget not all HIS benefits: WHO forgives all your iniquities, WHO heals all your diseases ..."

Psalms 107:20

"HE sent HIS word and healed them, And delivered them from their destructions."

Psalms 118:5-6

"I called on the LORD in distress; The LORD answered me and set me in a broad place. The LORD is on my side; I will not fear. What can man do to me?"

Proverbs 17:22

"A merry heart does good, like medicine, but a broken spirit dries the bones."

Ecclesiastes 3:3

"A time to heal; A time to break down, And a time to build up ..."

Isaiah 53:4-5

"Surely [Jesus][4] has borne our griefs And carried our sorrows; Yet we esteemed him stricken, Smitten by God, and afflicted. But [Jesus] was wounded for our transgressions, he was bruised for our iniquities; The chastisement for our peace was upon him, And by [the] stripes [of Jesus] we are healed."

Jeremiah 7:14

"Heal me, O LORD, and I shall be healed; Save me, and I shall be saved, For YOU [YAHWEH] are my praise."

Jeremiah 30:17

"For I will restore health to you and heal you of your wounds, says the LORD [God, YAHWEH, FATHER] ... "

Jeremiah 33:6

"Behold, I will bring [this place] health and healing; I will heal them and reveal to them the abundance of peace and truth."

Malachi 4:2

"But to you who fear MY name [YAHWEH] The Sun of Righteousness shall arise with healing in his wings; and you shall go out and grow fat like stall-fed calves."

Matthew 8:17

"... that it might be fulfilled, which was spoken by Isaiah the prophet, saying: "[Jesus] himself took our infirmities and bore our sicknesses."

Matthew 10:1-8

"And when [Jesus] had called his twelve disciples to him, [Jesus] gave them [delegated God's][5] power over unclean spirits, to cast them out, and to heal all kinds of sickness and all kinds of disease. ... These twelve Jesus sent out and commanded them, saying: 'Do not go into the way of the Gentiles, and do not enter a city of the Samaritans. But go rather to the lost sheep of the house of Israel. And as you go, preach, saying, The kingdom of heaven is at hand. Heal the sick, cleanse the lepers, raise the dead, cast out demons. Freely you have received, freely give.' "

Matthew 18:18-19

"Assuredly, I say to you, whatever you bind on earth will be bound in heaven, and whatever you loose on earth will be loosed in heaven. Again I say to you that if two of you agree on earth concerning anything that they ask, it will be done for them by my FATHER in heaven. For where two or three are gathered together in [Jesus'] name, I am there in the midst of them."

Mark 10:52

"Then Jesus said to him, 'Go your way; your faith has made you well.' And immediately he received his sight and followed Jesus on the road."

Mark 16:17-18

"And these signs will follow those who believe: In my [Jesus'] name they will cast out demons; they will speak with new tongues; they will take up serpents; and if they drink anything deadly, it will by no means hurt them; **they will lay hands on the sick, and they will recover.**"

Luke 5:17 (NAB)[6]

"One day as Jesus was teaching, Pharisees and teachers of the law were sitting there who had come from every village of Galilee and Judea and Jerusalem, and the power of the LORD [God, YAHWEH, FATHER] was with [Jesus] for healing."

Luke 8:50

"But when Jesus heard it, he answered him, saying, 'Do not be afraid; only believe, and she will be made well.' "

Luke 10:19

"Behold, I give you the authority to trample on serpents and scorpions, and over all the power of the enemy, and

nothing shall by any means hurt you."

Luke 17:18-19

"Were there not any found who returned to give glory to God except this foreigner? And [Jesus] said to him, "Arise, go your way. Your faith has made you well.""

Acts 9:33-34

"There he found a certain man named Aeneas, who had been bedridden eight years and was paralyzed. And Peter said to him, "Aeneas, Jesus the Christ heals you[7]. Arise and make your bed." Then he arose immediately.""

Romans 8:11

"But if the Spirit of HIM who raised Jesus from the dead dwells in you, HE who raised Christ from the dead will also give life to your mortal bodies through HIS Spirit who dwells in you."

James 5:16

"Confess your trespasses to one another, and pray for one another, that you may be healed. The effective, fervent prayer of a righteous man avails much."

James 5:14-16

"Is anyone among you sick? Let him call for the elders of

the church, and let them pray over him, anointing him with oil in the name of the [Jesus][8]. And the prayer of faith will save the sick, and the LORD[9] will raise him up. And if he has committed sins, he will be forgiven. Confess your trespasses to one another, and pray for one another, that you may be healed. The effective, fervent prayer of a righteous man avails much."

1 Peter 2:24
"[Jesus] who himself bore our sins in his own body on the tree, that we, having died to sins, might live for [God's] righteousness--by whose [Jesus] stripes you were healed."

Prayer Instructions

Some might argue that these verses were spoken to specific people or groups in the Bible and cannot be used personally for your healing. Your prayer task is to ignore such debates and focus on the principles shown. Then, understand that Jesus, the Apostles, and other strong prayer warriors are like an extension cord plugged into God's spiritual power plant. They are symbolically plugged into a spiritual power outlet, representing the Spirit power of YAHWEH, our living God. Therefore, it is not Jesus or they who heals you. Your healing comes from God through the hands or prayers of the firm believer [like Jesus] in the FATHER, our God, according to Jesus in John 20:17. That is why we pray to the FATHER and end our prayers "in the name of Jesus." Once you realize that God is your healer, you can use all these healing verses to get right with HIM and obtain HIS healing. You, too, can become a firm believer in the God Jesus believed in and prayed to for healing. Emulate Jesus!

In the case of a bad habit against someone's own body, it is not generally a sin that leads to immediate death. It is usually a slow killer of our own body. It is like the mythical story of a frog placed in a pan of cold water. According to the story, the frog will ignore what is happening when the water is slowly heated and eventually gets cooked alive. It could prevent its death if it were more intelligent and in tune, paying attention to its body. The story illustrates what happens in our bodies while engaging in bad health habits. Still, many are unable to stop their bad habits. Like the mythical frog, we think nothing is amiss with how we live our lives. We are wrong.

In our teens and twenties, we get away with beating our bodies pretty severely with a variety of unhealthy habits. As we get into our thirties, we then observe that some of our health habits are a cause of physical pain.

Maybe it is something small like the Italian hot sauce we always liked but no longer tolerable by our stomach? Perhaps it is that persistent cough that we realize is most likely linked to our smoking or vaping habit?

Maybe it is the slow increase in the quantity of alcoholic drinks because we no longer get a buzz very quickly. Now, we need 3-4 drinks, instead of the 1-2 we used to have at night. Yes, our body is building up a tolerance to alcohol poisoning. If we don't change our lousy health habit(s) by the time we are in the mid-forties, we reach the payback time. Verily, I say to you that I bear witness to many premature deaths beginning at age 45 linked directly to lousy health habits established early in life against the body. Two cousins drank themselves to death with alcohol at the age of 45. The second one mixed his alcohol with marijuana. Absolutely, this was not God's plan!

Think Habits, Change Habits!

We like to think we are an island unto ourselves. What we do is our own business. Right? Wrong! What we do affects everyone we love. If your bad health habits lead to a premature death, you deprive your children and grandchildren of precious love. It is evident in God's Word that your body is His temple. Once you begin to walk in His light, God owns a part of your flesh. It is also apparent in God's Word that, as husband or wife, we own a part of each other's bodies.

Therefore, if you are married and claim to walk with God and abuse your body with unhealthy habits, you also abuse a body that belongs to both God and your spouse. Thinking habits and changing habits was good advice I learned decades ago. The truth of that maxim still reigns.

Listen To Your Body

"Listen to what your body tells you" is also true. As we age, our bodies change. Suppose we don't alter calorie intake as we get into the thirties. In that case, the excess calories our bodies no longer need will be expressed on our bellies, thighs, or hips. The truth is our bodies are in a constant state of change. Literally, billions of cells die each day inside our bodies, and new cells are created. If you learn what happens at the cellular level of the body each day, it will astound you. When we are young, our calorie needs are more significant. As we age, caloric needs decline.

The body requires more attention as we age. Learn to listen to what your body is trying to tell you. Learn to alter your habits to improve your own physical health.

What is the best insurance policy you can own? Knowing you are a temple of the living God, where you are also the caretaker. Know what a precious gift your body is and learn how to properly take care of it.

My advice to you is to dump your bad health habits before they become a factor in your need for healing. And don't bother praying for the healing of your lungs if you are unwilling to stop smoking. Don't bother praying for your diseased liver if you are a chronic alcoholic who refuses to stop drinking. Don't tell me that you can't stop. I know for a fact that you will eventually stop.

The big question is whether you will have the courage to help yourself before it is too late. You can pray for God's help to give you the wisdom and the courage to change or quit. God does expect you to exert some common sense over the health issues affecting your body. It is because God has built into your body some fantastic healing powers on a cellular level. HE has also given you the spirit of a strong mind. This means that you have a direct role in your healing. Accepting that fact means you'll understand God's self-care[10] medical health plan.

However, it would help if you exerted willpower to change your bad habits. No one can do it for you. If your bad health habits lead to your premature death, you only have yourself to blame. Systematically killing your own body is not God's plan. HIS plan is for a natural death at

HIS appointed time. Likewise, the 11-year-old boy who was killed while picking up the family's mail had his life cut short by an adult driver exercising her 66-year-old free will. Killing that boy with her car was not God's plan.

To the extent your free will intersects with another's, and it results in their premature death, it is not the plan of God ALMIGHTY! HIS plan is defined in Genesis[11], in which HE says we can live to be 120 years old, and in Jeremiah, where a future with hope is promised. Of course, this assumes you are more intelligent than the mythical frog and are also not the victim of being accidentally or intentionally killed by another human.

"For I know the plans I have for you, says the LORD. They are plans for good and not for disaster, to give you a future and a hope." Jeremiah 29:11 NLT

Don't blame all the evil in this earth on God ALMIGHTY. Man's sin, free will, ignorance, and errant ways are responsible for a lot of it, and the balance of the evil is Satan at work. Aside from the long life and future of hope, God also provides us with good things. That is God's nature.

"Every good gift and every perfect gift is from

above, and comes down from the FATHER of lights, with whom there is no variation or shadow of turning." James 1:17

"And we know that all things work together for good to those who love God, to those who are the called according to HIS purpose." Romans 8:28

Life As God Designed Means

We Have A Responsibility For Our Own Heath!

So we can cut short or lengthen our life span by bad or good health habits. Our lives can also be cut short by events of other people that are beyond our control. In both cases, if life ends prematurely, it does not end by God's design. God's plan was to have us reach our "appointed time." Now, let's examine some graphics.

Before the funeral of the 11-year-old son of my friend Connie, God gave me three illustrations to explain why some deaths are not at HIS appointed time. First, we can imagine that in God's design, our spirit souls would move smoothly through life in the right direction, peacefully coexisting with all other souls.

This is represented in the graphic below, showing

seven lines with arrows pointing to the right. Each line is representative of a spirit soul on this earth. The loops around the individual spirit souls represent one or more groups of spirit souls that fellowship and share life together. People might belong to more than one group, and in this way, our society grows by sharing life with each other. Sometimes, loners like to stay to themselves [bottom arrow]. In God's design, we all get along without conflict, moving from left to right [**arrow heads** indicate life direction]. Now enters sin.

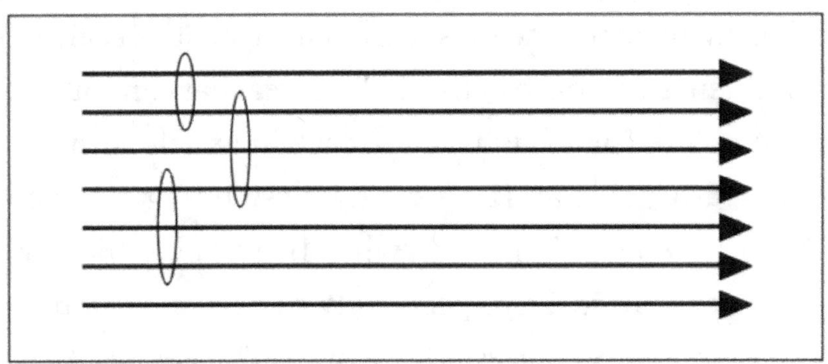

The Spirit-Soul Life As God Designed

God's perfect plan did not unfold as HE intended once man had sinned and the knowledge of evil entered man's thoughts. You may have learned that Satan is the winner of the massive amount of spirit souls on this earth. What happened in Noah's time is set to happen once again. Few follow the narrow path and are saved according to

Jesus. As a direct result of the knowledge of evil, this world belongs to Satan [at least temporarily], and we do live in a life of literal chaos. Instead of all spirit souls moving in the "right" direction as God had intended, some move all over the place, crisscrossing one another and, in essence, crashing into one another. This causes many contentions. See the following graphic.

All the **arrows** that move in a direction not intended by God [left to right] represent the chaos in this earthly life that confronts our spirit souls. The **dots** are areas of conflict because of opposing human forces at work. It explains why someone dies a premature death because of the influence of a destructive habit force that cannot be overcome. It explains why a 66-year-old female drunk driver crashes into an 11-year-old boy standing at the end of his driveway and kills him while he retrieves the mail.

We were supposed to peacefully coexist, live a long life, and then die a natural death at God's appointed time. However, all bets are off unless we get close to God and take advantage of His protection to the maximum degree possible. God will protect His people, but remember that He has a bigger picture. We have only limited visibility of His plans. God also gave humanity free will, which means we all make our own life choices.

Sometimes, our choices in life collide with the choices of other people. The intersection of individual human

God And Cancer: A Self-Care Perspective

choices [**dots**] shows areas of conflict, physical harm, and chaos caused by human behavior. For the most part, the chaos in this earthly life directly results from human choices or the conflict posed by the intersection of two or more human decisions. Life's chaos is an expression of human free will.

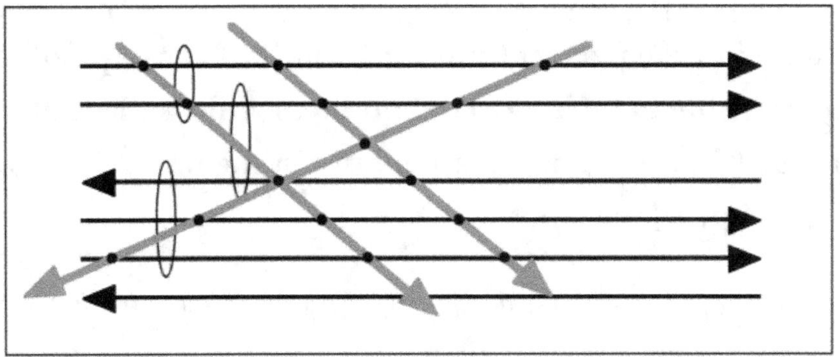

The Spirit-Soul Life In Satan's World

When God says HIS grace is sufficient--you will never fully understand why. Like Paul and myself, where healing did not result from prayers, it may be a bitter pill to swallow. Yet God knows what is best for us, and our understanding will be fulfilled when we see our LORD and HIS Son. For now, ponder the graphic above and try to understand that we live in a world that we were never supposed to live in. It is a world of evil desires and works of the flesh that conflict with God's ways. God has drawn a line down the middle of all cultures; choose a side. Suffering will increase worldwide as sin increases, morals sink further, and societal lawlessness continues unabated. See the following graphic.

We read the following from the Gnostic Gospel of Philip[12] concerning God's protection of sincere believers.

"The [evil] powers[13] do not see those who are clothed in the perfect light [of God], and consequently are not able to [affect or] detain them. One will clothe himself in this light sacramentally in the union[14] [with God's Spirit]." See notes.

For years, I have felt God's protection in my life. An unusual feeling of security moves with you wherever you go. Listen to some Bible verses that speak of the protection that God provides.

Satan said: "Have YOU not made a hedge [of protection] around him, around his household, and around all that he has on every side? YOU have blessed the work of his hands, and his possessions have increased in the land." Job 1:10

Jesus said: "I do not pray that YOU [FATHER] should take them out of the world, but that YOU should keep them from the evil one [and protect them]." John 17:15

"For HE shall give HIS angels charge over you, to [protect you and] keep you in all your ways." Psalm 91:11

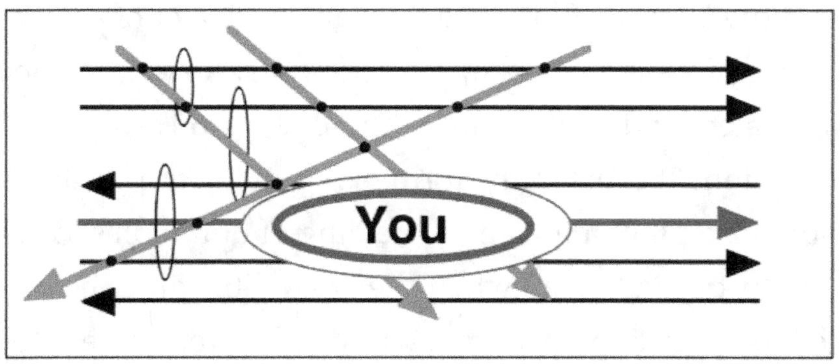

You In Satan's World With Holy Spirit

It is possible to move through this world with a high degree of God's protection. The graphic above shows a hedge of protection that surrounds God's servant. Think of it as a force field that can deflect the evil of this world so that its full impact is not felt. It is the result of putting on the whole armor of God. I have seen many examples of God's protection[15].

Some time ago, my adopted granddaughter Amy survived a near-fatal car accident, which the state patrol officer said was unbelievable and almost 100% fatal. Her car was hit head-on by a drunk driver driving down the interstate highway in the wrong direction. The rescue workers had to literally cut her out of the vehicle with machines[16].

The femur bone on each leg was broken in two, and she had to have them pinned and screwed together. She was only 20 years old at the time and had a lot of other physical damage. I am happy to report she is doing fine, has healed, and walks again. Where was God's protection? It came in the form of surviving the crash. Youth also plays a role in the healing of our bodies. Amy and I lost a big toenail when she was a little girl. She grew hers back in only three weeks. Mine took a year to grow back. As we age, the length of our years becomes a factor in healing; make no mistake.

God offered similar protection for Jesus and his disciples. It often came as survival or getting out of the way just in time. It usually involved pain and suffering, too. Study Paul's travels for some classic illustrations of trouble coupled with divine protection.

When my grandson Braiden was nine months old, he choked on a bottle-cap-sized chunk of jagged glass at the back of his throat. My daughter-in-law managed to get it out. To our amazement, Braiden did not have as much as a scratch. We believe that this was divine protection and an answer to our prayers. We ask God for the protection of our family every time we pray, and we have seen many such miracles.

Healing is a sticky point for many Christians who assert that God always heals. Usually, there is a caveat indicating that, of course, it depends upon one's faith. However, all bets are off if there is sin in your life. Does the Word teach us that healing always comes from prayer?

Suppose momentarily that a Charismatic fellow claims that God will always heal him. To illustrate the point, he jumps out in front of a semi-truck with 18 wheels and gets mangled. After months in the hospital and two years of physical therapy, he says to you that it proves he was right. I'll tell you what it proves. It proves he was stupid and that God was gracious. When he says he can do it again to prove the truth of the point, do you think he has much upstairs in the brain department? If he does jump in front of another truck, do you believe God will still be gracious and heal him? God's grace is at the center of all divine healing.

Jesus told them, "When you pray, say YOUR [YAHWEH, God ALMIGHTY, FATHER] will be done on earth as it is in Heaven." Luke 11:2

Prayer: LORD, *teach us to understand* YOUR *sovereignty, grace, and mercy. Teach us to pray as Jesus did and seek* YOUR *will, not ours.*

The story of King David further illustrates Divine healing. David fasted and prayed while his son was stricken. In the end, the child died. When asked why he stopped grieving, he gives us an enlightening illustration of God's sovereignty. Go back and study this lack of healing in 2 Samuel 12:21-23 despite the sincere prayer of King David.

Therefore, between King David and King Hezekiah, we have both situations regarding healing due to prayer. In one case, healing was denied, and in the other, healing took place. But in both cases, it was the grace of God.

David and Hezekiah acknowledged God's sovereignty over their life and death. Do you? If not, death will not make much sense to you, and your suffering will continue unabated when a loved one suddenly dies. You will not understand like King David and I do that you too will go to see your loved one someday, but that your loved one will not come back to earth to see you.

CHAPTER NINE
Jesus Always Healed?

But Edward, you say, Jesus always healed people! I would reply: "You are misinformed of biblical facts." Consider the following Bible verses if you think Jesus always healed every one.

"Now he did not do many mighty works there because of their unbelief." Matthew 13:55-58 NKJV

"And he did not do many miracles there because of their unbelief." Matthew 13:58 NASB

"And he did not work many miracles there because of their lack of faith." Matthew 13:58 NJB

"He didn't work many miracles there because of their lack of faith." Matthew 13:58 GW

Here is the full context from the NLT translation.

" 'He's just a carpenter's son, and we know Mary, his mother, and his brothers-James, Joseph, Simon, and Judas. All his sisters live right here among us. What makes him so great?' And they were deeply offended and refused to believe in him. Then Jesus told them, 'A prophet is honored everywhere except in his own hometown and among his own family.' And so he did only a few miracles there because of their unbelief." Matthew 13:55-58 NLT

I heard a radio preacher illustrate this verse in which he proclaimed: "God refused to do miracles in His hometown because of their lack of faith." *Note the confusion of who Jesus is.* His teaching was that God chose not to do miracles in His hometown. The interpretation is an error. The correct reading should be that Jesus [not God] could not do even more miracles because of the lack of faith in his [Jesus'] hometown. You can learn two things from this verse. First of all, Jesus did not heal everyone. At least he did not in his hometown because that much is implicit. Secondly, our individual and even collective faith plays a role in our healing.

Jesus asks the poignant question: "Do you want to be healed?"

"When Jesus saw him lying there, and knew that he already had been in that condition a long time, he said to him, 'Do you want to be made well?' " John 5:6

Personal Desire & Will Power Matters To God!

Our faith or lack of faith plays a vital role in healing. Jesus gives us many illustrations where faith was a direct attribute in achieving miraculous healing. However, personal desire for healing and individual willpower also play a role. Isn't that why Jesus asked: "Do you want to be healed?" The plain truth is that many people do not want to be healed but would not openly say that to loved ones.

Some people with long-term disabilities want to continue to live in misery because, unbelievably, they have come to look forward to the attention and pity of others. They have also grown accustomed to some meager expectations for their life. Yet many other people want to move on to their heavenly home. They are put out about this earthly life. Some even feel the "pull" from the heavenly side is much stronger than the "pull" from this earthly side. Simply put, they want to check out as naturally as possible in God's eyes.

I had the chance to talk to a banking acquaintance

named Carolyn. At one time, we had attended the same church. A mutual friend told me that she had cancer and only had a short time to live. God told me to call her and tell her about the nutritional supplements that I had uncovered for healing cancer at the cellular level. There are, surprisingly, many natural cures available for cancer that are being stifled and kept hidden from the public's view by the allopathic medical industry. Perhaps Carolyn could use some of them, even though we had limited success with my wife?

As it turned out, Carolyn was not interested in any potential cancer cures on the cellular level. She had a strong faith and was intent on moving on. In fact, she told me that the heavenly pull was much stronger for her than anything on this earth. That included her family. She told me she was trying to prepare the family so they would understand. It sounded like the family wanted her to undergo various treatment options, which she was soundly rejecting. She was ready for the heavenly mansion she knew was already prepared for her.

Virtually everyone older than my first wife and me on both sides of the family has already died and moved on. My first wife also looked forward to moving on, and this was an undeniable attribute that impacted her healing. When my small church group laid hands on her, she said the magical words "Thank You, Jesus." That night, she began to arise again. The following two weeks were astonishing to me. God had touched her body that night, and we all knew it. Yet, it turned out to be the last gasp of energy that flowed out of her body. Still, I enjoyed watching my wife have some fun once again.

Pray earnestly in great faith for your own healing. There is no doubt this helps. You can even wear sackcloth and fast like many biblical people did during sickness and grieving. Yet there is still the sovereignty issue of God's graciousness and mercy, as explained by Moses, King David, and Apostle Paul.

Come to God with a loyal heart, having walked by His definition of righteousness. That is my best advice to you in these matters where divine healing is needed and sought. Get as close to God as you can. True faith begins by accepting the reality in our hearts that we do serve a living God. Here are more verses where faith is an attribute.

Strong Faith & A Loyal Heart Matter To God!

"But Jesus turned around, and when he saw her he said, 'Be of good cheer, daughter; your faith has made you well.' And the woman was made well from that hour." Matthew 9:22

"Then he [Jesus]touched their eyes, saying, 'According to your faith let it be to you.' " Matthew 9:29

"Then Jesus answered and said to her, 'O woman, great is your faith! Let it be to you as you desire.' And her daughter was healed from that very hour." Matthew 15:28

"Then Jesus said to him, 'Go your way; your faith has made you well.' And immediately he received his sight and followed Jesus on the road." Mark 10:52

It is not just your faith that matters when it comes to healing prayer. God clarifies that those who pray for you can influence the outcome. Therefore, join your faith with others who trust God for the desired result. Again, this doesn't always get you what you want. However, it will surely come true if you ask anything according to God's will.

"Now this is the confidence that we have in HIM, that if we ask anything according to HIS will, HE hears us. And if we know that HE hears us, whatever we ask, we know that we have the petitions that we have asked of HIM." 1 John 5:14-15

Likewise, it will not come true if you ask anything that is not God's will.

"You ask and do not receive, because you ask amiss." James 4:3

What should you do when you are sick? Follow James' instructions.

"Is anyone among you sick? Let him [this is you] call for the elders [prayer warriors] of the church, and let them pray over him, anointing him with oil in the name of the LORD. And the prayer of faith will save the sick, and the LORD will raise him up. And if he has committed sins, he will be forgiven." James 5:14-15

"Confess your trespasses to one another, and pray for one another, that you may be healed. The effective, fervent prayer of a righteous man avails much." James 5:16

A Prayer Of Faith
Will Save The Sick!

Your healing goal in terms of prayer should be to get

into a practical and fervent prayer. This should be with one or more righteous persons whose hearts are loyal to God. Many who read the above verses would say that they prove God will heal us. I cannot emphasize a singular fact enough. You cannot lift single verses out of the context of the entire Bible. To do so ignores God's bigger picture and His eternal character. You cannot assume that God will heal you unless you will also recognize His sovereignty over your life and that He might not heal you. Your job is to exercise your faith to the best of your ability and then put your fate into the hands of God Almighty. Having done all, stand on faith.

"Therefore take up the whole armor of God, that you may be able to withstand in the evil day, and having done all, to stand." Ephesians 6:13

I have witnessed both wild successes and sad disappointments in divine healing. I can never really say why healing comes to some and why it doesn't come to others, except for God's bigger picture. I say this because I have witnessed the strength of powerful prayer in both of these outcomes. Therefore, I know that the prayer of faith was answered in some cases and not others.

To my young friends at a Charismatic church that claims God will always heal, I say: "Go check and find out how many people died in your 10,000-member church this last year, and come tell me the same thing."

If God had always healed, we would not have suffered so many losses each year within the Church despite many solid prayers of faith. Honest prayers of faith are made like how Jesus taught us to pray. Jesus taught us to pray that God's will should be done.

Ultimately, God is not a slot machine whereby one makes a demand upon the anointing and gets what they want. That is the stuff of Christian mythology in the "name it and claim it" crowd[1]. Genuine, sincere faith will yield to God in every situation, and we are taught nothing less than that in the Holy Bible Christians profess to believe in. This doesn't mean you should not exercise your faith. It is the opposite: exercise your faith and trust in God to deal with the outcome.

What should you do to pray for someone if you get that subtle message inside? You should pray regardless of the time of day or night you get that unction from God's Spirit. Your prayer may make the difference between life and death. What should you do if you get the message to go to a hospital or nursing home to pray for someone? Get up and go and pray for them, even if you do not know why. Too many people ignore the unction of the Holy Spirit in their lives. It is one reason our families suffer needlessly in this life. Here are some prayer examples.

A Healed Heart

Our family's friend, Kathryn, was purging her food with an over-the-counter syrup used to induce vomiting. She had bulimia. By the time we learned of the problem, she crashed and was on her deathbed in the hospital. Her heart had expanded physically to four times its standard size as a result of her eating disorder and uncontrolled lousy habits. She was placed on a heart machine for a more extended period than anyone in history; she was given less than a 5% chance of survival when the machine was removed. Our family mounted a prayer vigil at the hospital and spoke healing over her body using some of the verses shown earlier. Eventually, she was healed and is an example to others about her eating disorder. It was divine healing, and no one can deny what had happened to her and how God intervened to save her life.

Legs Untouched

Prayer for my dear friend's wife was met with virtually no change. She is still restricted to a wheelchair, and both legs are still totally dysfunctional.

Wheel Chairs Untouched

My personal observation is that people in wheelchairs usually remain there if it has been many years. I have never witnessed physically reconstructive healing, such as spinal regeneration or the growth of new bones, etc. We know that this kind of healing did occur in the Bible. Therefore, I believe in such healings and have often thrown my faith into prayer. I have witnessed only those whose bodies were deathly sick healed by the prayer of faith as the Apostle James taught. Why healing occurs in some cases and not in others may be related to God's glory, as Jesus explains.

Jesus said: "Go and tell John the things which you hear and see: The blind see and the lame walk; the lepers are cleansed and the deaf hear; the dead are raised up and the poor have the gospel preached to them." Matthew 11:4-5

"As Jesus was walking along, he saw a man who had been blind from birth. 'Teacher,' his disciples asked him, 'why was this man born blind? Was it a result of his own sins or those of his parents?' 'It was not because of his sins or his parents' sins,' Jesus answered.

'He was born blind so the power of God could be seen in him.' " John 9:1-3 NLT

Sometimes, a severe physical abnormality exists in people simply so God's power can be seen in that person. It is a witness to all when someone who suffers physical limitations can still magnify God. Their faith is a massive testimony because of their physical limitations. Many blind people can do things that those with sight cannot do. Many lame can do things the physically able cannot do. I know of blind people who play music even though they cannot read music sheets. I know of people without arms who play guitars with their feet. Many such examples can be illustrated. How does this happen? It is accomplished through faith in God, and all of the success of the disabled is a living testimony to the non-disabled that God does exist and inspires people to lead remarkable lives despite severe limitations.

It is a sad commentary that the non-disabled often cannot deal with bad health habits. At the same time, severely disabled people accomplish such wondrous things.

CHAPTER TEN
Death Cheated

I remember the moment I got the message to go down to the hospital and lay hands on my good friend Al for his healing. I can't recall that I had ever laid hands on someone who was on a deathbed before. Al was close to death from hepatitis destroying his liver. My son-in-law James, a man of similar faith, worked with me then. I told him, "James, God gave me the message to go down tonight and pray for Al. Do you want to come with me?" James responded, "I got the same message, what time do you want to go?"

It is simple: the Spirit of YAHWEH spoke within us, as Jesus explained. Get used to listening to HIS sweet, soft voice and learn to understand when HE speaks in you. If it is good, makes complete sense, and aligns with God's Word, you can be confident that the voice you hear inside your mind is from God.

"Do not worry about how or what you should speak. For it will be given to you in that hour what you should

speak; for it is not you who speak, but the Spirit of your FATHER [YAHWEH] who speaks in you." Matthew 10:19-20

By the time James and I arrived at the isolation ward that Al was in, he was looking pretty bad. His skin was darkened as if he had been sunbathing for months, and his eyes were yellow. There was little doubt his body was stricken with a deadly disease. Al explained that he was unable to move much and was very weak. He could barely lift his arm. I asked if his parish priest had touched his body for divine healing. Al explained that the priest had been there three times and prayed.

I ascertained from the conversation that no one had touched him for healing, even though many had prayed for him for several weeks. I knew we would be deep into the Spirit as we laid hands on him and prayed; it meant speaking in tongues. I told Al that he would understand that hands had been laid on him for DIVINE healing when we were done. I also told him to ignore what we were doing or saying. I said: "Close your eyes, Al, and simply reach out and grab the healing God wants you to have. Thank God for your healing because it is not your time to die."

I started the prayer, and James and I altered praying in and out of tongues for Al's healing for about twenty minutes. I still remember God's incredible presence in that hospital room. All I could see in my spirit were bright lights and fireworks. Ultimately, God gave my spirit total satisfaction that healing was done. I told James it was time to go. God healed Al, and he was up and shaving in only a few hours and moving for the first time in days. But there are more fantastic parts of the story.

Earlier that very day, Al underwent another liver test. The results this time showed his liver needed a transplant. It was no longer functioning. As the doctor came into the room to give Al the bad news, he found Al sitting upright in a chair, looking revived from death. Once again, a medical doctor was left befuddled.

Death Cheated Temporarily

It was a few years later that my sister Barb wound up in the ICU ward of a hospital in northern Minnesota after a scheduled surgery went awry. When my brother and I got the message of her condition, she was near death. We decided to go up and lay hands on her for healing. I was terrified then that my faith would not be good enough. This time, I was so emotional and in tears over her impending death that I did not even know if I could pray a "prayer of faith." I was shaken. I asked James to come with his faith.

By the time we got to Barb's ICU room, the death rattle was already on her body. Her kidneys had both stopped functioning for days, and her lungs were now almost filled up with fluid. Death was imminent, and there was little doubt about it. As we prayed, I was not given all the input from God during Al's healing prayer. We returned to her home for the night, placing her firmly into God's loving hands.

When we returned to the hospital the following day, both kidneys had started working again, and Barb's lungs were clear. I was stunned. I asked the nurse when her lungs had cleared up. The attending nurse didn't have any answers. While she was in the hospital, it was my privilege to pray with her to receive the Holy Spirit. I watched Barb recover and go home. It allowed me to visit with her at length and let her know how much I loved her and what she had meant to me in this life. We were able to share a lot.

I remember the last time I visited with her. She explained how much pain she was in, and I told her to give everything over to God. That night, as she lay in bed and I was studying in her living room, I remember hearing her cry out in pain to God for relief. It was a heart-breaking cry from the bowels of Barb's soul. She screamed out loud: "Oh God, please help me!" I remember joining with her in a prayer for God to heal her hurting body. Barb died about three months after we resurrected her body from death in the ICU ward. I will always be grateful for the extra time that God gave me with her. When she died, I knew it was her time. God honored the family by giving us time to share and say our final goodbyes.

Of course, there are many more details to the events I relate to you in this chapter. If I had tried to cover all of them, each event would have been worthy of its own book. As a result of these experiences, God gave me a simple formula for His divine healing. Take it to heart. In addition, God gave me the following illustration of Jesus' prayer.

Prayer of Faith = Belief in Healing + Trust in God's Bigger Picture

When you exercise your "prayer of faith," the two ingredients you need are a genuine belief that God will heal someone and a trust that if God does not, it is because of His bigger picture. I mention this as Christianity has different levels of faith and belief. You must act in faith "as if" God will deliver your loved one's healing. Many people do not believe in divine healing today. There are even people who do not believe in the resurrection.

Unbelievable for Christians in both cases, but they do exist. Do not bring someone into the "prayer of faith" who does not believe in divine healing. If you do, they can literally "suck" the spiritual energy out of the prayer. It is better to have people who believe totally in healing than "anyone" who doesn't believe in healing but thinks the prayer motions are good therapy for the family.

Employ God's "As-If" Principle
In "Prayers Of Faith!"

The power of your prayers is enhanced when you deploy the biblical "as-if principle" explained by Paul in Romans 4. You envision the healing that God is delivering in your mind and spirit. That is to say that you do not see things as the world sees them. You know that two realities exist. One is the reality our senses detect; the other is God's reality. In God's spiritual realm, HE calls things into existence that did not exist before. In the present case, healing. Therefore, be like God and call healing into existence.

"This happened because Abraham believed in the God who brings the dead back to life and who brings into existence what didn't exist before." Rom. 4:17 NLT

I flipped through two old, tattered, and marked-up Bibles to find the "as-if" principle. Norman Vincent Peale taught it to me several decades ago. It works in all areas of life in situations where God doesn't have another plan for you. Regardless of what your senses tell you, you should never stop praying. Sometimes, the nature of prayer might change like mine did with my father-in-law, who died of colon cancer. We prayed earnestly for healing for many months.

However, his body became severely emaciated, and his pain became intolerable. Eventually, the nature of our prayers changed. God showed me that it was time for me to pray for mercy. That is what we then prayed for. We also told him that it was okay to go home. In the realm of dying and "shedding our flesh," it can become evident that healing is not in God's bigger picture. Remember, God does not need months or years to heal someone.

When you realize the need for mercy, you must also spiritually release your loved one. More than one person has endured suffering because they were afraid to leave a loved one who was clinging to them emotionally. A lack of a family member's emotional and spiritual release of their dying loved one unnecessarily held them in their body on this earthly plane. In many cases, it resulted in a delayed death and an extended period of horrific pain.

Listen. Do not unduly hold your loved ones on this

earthly plain. To do so increases their pain and suffering. It is a very self-centered thing, and Christ teaches us not to live for ourselves. As a father or mother needs to give their child wings to leave the house, we all need to give our dying family members their wings to go home. My daughter asked Connie: "Do you know what to say when someone asks how many kids you have?" Connie said no. Patty replied: "Tell them you have two that can walk and one that can fly." She knows what it means to let go.

Jesus Said: "Always Pray & Do Not Lose Heart!"

"Then [Jesus] spoke a parable to them, that men [or women] always ought to pray and not lose heart." Luke 18:1

Your spiritual understanding should include the complete Word of God and not just narrow sections or single verses of the Bible. God's bigger context is HIS entire Word. That is why the healing Jesus discussed in Matthew 9:35 does not apply to Nazareth. God's Word teaches us something different about Jesus' hometown. The miracles of Jesus were done at the direction of YAHWEH. Therefore, pray to YAHWEH, your God, just like Jesus did. Realize, like Jesus did, that not all prayers are answered as we want them to be.

"When things go well, be glad; but when they go ill, consider this: God has set the one alongside the other in such a way that no one can find out what is to happen afterwards [next]." Ecclesiastes 7:14 REB

Spiritual translation
You never know what life will bring next!

Jesus did not want to leave us. He did not want to die on that cross, and his prayer to God reflected that clear thought in his mind. His willingness to do so resulted from his love for YAHWEH [his FATHER and God]. Listen to a prayer from Jesus that was not answered the way he wanted. If God did not answer all of Jesus' prayers in the way he wanted, why should you be surprised if some of your prayers are not answered how you want them to?

Jesus said: "Abba, FATHER, all things are possible for YOU. Take this cup away from me; nevertheless, not what I will, but what YOU will." Mark 14:36

Are you willing to yield to God's will just like Jesus Christ? If not, why? Are you not supposed to follow the example of Christ?

PART TWO

DIY Healing Your Body

CHAPTER ELEVEN
Water & Healing

I used to think that water was simple enough for everyone to understand. After all, it is H20, which has one hydrogen atom, two oxygen atoms, and three phases, right? Liquid, solid, and steam, correct? Well, water is more complex now. Water is so complex that scientists no longer fully understand everything about water. To start with, scientists now know that there are four phases of water. Add a jello-like state to the other three widely known states of water.

Our bodies are 60-75% water, and most surround our cells. Scientists are discovering that water can communicate, and some now believe that water may be responsible for intercellular communications. They also found that water has electrical properties[1], which scientists are studying.

For healing, with all we currently know, unless you keep your body hydrated, you are subjecting your body to a host of various diseases and metabolic complications. In contrast, you can drown yourself by drinking too much water. Pinching the skin on the top of your hand and seeing how fast it goes back to normal is one way of determining if you are hydrated. Another way is to observe the color of your urine. A body needing hydrating will exhibit a very dark color in its urine. An adequately hydrated body will have clear urine. That is true unless the person consumes vitamins, which can produce a light green or yellow appearance. Foods such as asparagus and beets can also color urine.

Dehydration

Dehydration is a risk factor for various chronic diseases, such as hypertension, cardiovascular diseases, diabetes, and kidney diseases. Staying hydrated can lower the risk of these conditions and improve their management.

In the case of hypertension, drinking enough water helps to lower blood pressure. When dehydrated, the body compensates by constricting blood vessels, increasing blood pressure. Adequate water intake helps maintain blood volume and prevent high blood pressure.

Water intake is also crucial for individuals with diabetes. Proper hydration can help regulate blood sugar levels, as it helps the kidneys eliminate excess glucose through urine. Additionally, drinking water before meals can promote a sense of fullness, leading to decreased food consumption and better blood sugar control.

Chronic kidney disease (CKD) is another condition that requires careful hydration. Water helps to maintain kidney function by flushing waste products from the body. Individuals with CKD should drink enough water to keep their urine light-colored and to prevent dehydration, which can worsen their kidney function.

Furthermore, water is essential for weight management, which is closely linked to chronic diseases such as obesity, heart disease, and certain types of cancer. Drinking water before meals helps to reduce calorie intake, promote weight loss, and prevent weight gain. It also boosts metabolism, aiding in the burning of calories.

Water is also crucial in managing digestive disorders, such as constipation. Constipation often occurs due to insufficient fiber intake and dehydration. Drinking enough water helps to soften the stool, making it easier to pass and alleviating constipation. You may already know about the health issues involved with water.

However, water can be essential in healing beyond just hydrating the body. What this section will reveal to you are the other ways that water can assist in healing your body. I will explain the following six additional water qualities that can affect healing, which you might not know but need to understand. That is especially true if you are now fighting cancer[2] in your body. I'm assuming you want to live and get rid of the disease. If not, see my note because this discussion of water won't matter to you.

How Water Can Affect The Body

1) Oxidation
2) Water Oxidation
3) Molecular Hydrogen (H2) Water
4) Deuterium Depleted Water (DDW)
5) The Interstitium[3]
6) The Fascia[4]

Oxidation

The easiest way to understand oxidation is to cut an apple in half and expose it on the kitchen counter. In short order, the apple will start turning brown. That is a visible oxidation (brown-colored) caused by the apple's exposure to oxygen.

Oxidation is a normal metabolic process that occurs in the body. It involves the reaction of oxygen with various body molecules. Oxidation often leads to the formation of highly reactive molecules called free radicals. These are unstable atoms or molecules with unpaired electrons in their outer shells. Free radicals are generally unstable and highly reactive, seeking to stabilize themselves by "stealing" electrons from other molecules in the body, such as proteins, lipids, and DNA. This process is called oxidative stress.

While a certain level of free radicals is necessary for normal cellular functions, excessive and uncontrolled production of these molecules can cause damage to cells and tissues. Various health conditions, including aging, inflammation, cardiovascular diseases, neurodegenerative diseases like Alzheimer's and Parkinson's, and cancer, are linked to oxidative stress.

The body has built-in defense mechanisms in the form of antioxidants that counteract the harmful effects of oxidation. Antioxidants can neutralize and stabilize free radicals, preventing them from causing damage. Some antioxidants are produced naturally in the body. In contrast, others come from dietary sources, such as fruits, vegetables, certain spices, and nutraceuticals like Vitamin C supplementation.

Maintaining a balance between oxidation and antioxidation is essential for overall health and well-being. You can achieve this by adopting a healthy lifestyle, including a well-balanced diet rich in antioxidants, regular exercise, adequate sleep, and avoiding exposure to environmental toxins and excessive stress. Additionally, certain antioxidant supplements may be beneficial when natural antioxidant defenses are overwhelmed or compromised.

Grounding[5] mats, sheets, and other methods can give the body free electrons from the Earth to help neutralize free radicals and the damage they cause. The Earth has a negative charge and is an abundant source of free electrons via grounding (aka earthing). Grounding to the Earth allows free electrons from the Earth to function like that of antioxidants in the repair of free radicals within the body.

Water Oxidation

Water's oxidation ability is generally not harmful to the human body because water is a neutral molecule. However, water can facilitate oxidation reactions when other substances that can undergo oxidation are present and cause the formation of free radicals.

Water contaminated with certain chemicals or pollutants can also contribute to oxidative stress and harm the human body. For example, water containing heavy metals, pesticides, or other toxic substances can increase oxidative damage and lead to various health problems.

While water does not pose a direct risk due to its

oxidation ability, its role in facilitating oxidative reactions with other harmful substances can potentially harm the human body.

Alkaline water and Hydrogen-rich water can minimize oxidation in the body. Alkaline water has a higher pH level, which can act as an antioxidant and help neutralize free radicals in the body. Meanwhile, Hydrogen-rich water contains molecular Hydrogen (H2), which has antioxidant properties and can help reduce oxidative stress.

Your drinking water might be good or bad for your body. It may also contain higher levels of oxidation than you need to drink. Get some pH strips and check if your water is acidic or alkaline (typically a pH of 7.0 or higher[6]). That should be the first test of your water's quality. You can also measure the mineral and organic content of the water. That would be an excellent second test of your water's quality.

Minimize Water Oxidation

To minimize the oxidation properties of your drinking water, follow the following steps:

Choose the right water source: Use a high-quality water source low in minerals and organic matter, which can help reduce the water's oxidation potential.

Proper storage: Store water in a clean and tightly sealed container. Exposure to air and contaminants can increase oxidative properties. Consider using glass or stainless steel containers instead of plastic[7], as they are less likely to leach chemicals into the water.

Filter the water: Invest in a good quality water filter that can remove impurities and reduce the concentration of minerals and organic matter. Look for filters specifically designed to minimize oxidation potential.

Treat the water with antioxidants: Adding antioxidant substances to drinking water can help neutralize any potential oxidation. For example, you can add a few drops of lemon juice containing Vitamin C, a natural antioxidant. However, be cautious with the quantity, as too much lemon juice can alter the taste of water.

Avoid excessive exposure to air: When pouring water, try to do it gently to minimize contact with air. Rapid pouring and splashing can increase the water's oxidation potential.

Consume fresh water: It's preferable to consume relatively fresh water stored for only a short period. If you store water, replenish your supply regularly to maintain its quality.

Keep water away from sunlight: Exposure to sunlight can promote oxidation in water. Store the water in a dark and cool place, away from direct sunlight.

Use antioxidant supplements: Consider taking antioxidant supplements, such as Vitamins C and E, which can help minimize oxidative stress in your body. That can indirectly reduce the impact of any potential oxidation in drinking water.

Remember, while minimizing oxidation in drinking water can be beneficial, it is essential to maintain overall good water quality through regular testing and appropriate filtration methods.

Molecular Hydrogen (H2) Water

Hydrogen water is water infused with molecular Hydrogen (H2) gas. According to alternative health doctors, Hydrogen is a potent antioxidant with significant health benefits. These benefits include reducing inflammation, improving athletic performance, and promoting overall well-being.

There are several ways you can enhance the Hydrogen content of drinking water. I've used two low-cost and easy methods of adding molecular Hydrogen (H2) to my drinking water, which I discuss below. However, four primary methods are currently used to enhance water with molecular Hydrogen (H2) for health benefits.

Water ionizers: These machines use electrolysis to split the water into alkaline and acidic components, with the alkaline water containing molecular Hydrogen.

Hydrogen tablets or powders: Small tablets or powders can be dissolved in water to add molecular Hydrogen.

Hydrogen water generators: These devices have a chamber that produces Hydrogen gas, which is then dissolved into the water to create Hydrogen water.

Hydrogen water bottles: These portable bottles can infuse water with Hydrogen gas to create hydrogen-enhanced water on the go.

I have used H2 tablets dissolved in water. It is straightforward to use. You drop an H2 tablet into 16 ounces of water and let it dissolve. The tablet is effervescent and will dissolve in 2-5 minutes. Once dissolved, the Hydrogen gas can evaporate fast, so you need to drink the water immediately, within 5-10 minutes after the tablet dissolves. While I've usually done this in the morning while consuming vitamins, one doctor recommends doing this before bed for additional health benefits. It is a relatively inexpensive way to improve your health. I have certainly noticed improved energy from drinking molecular hydrogen-enhanced water. You can find molecular Hydrogen (H2) products here[8]. See notes for the links to the two H2 products I have used.

The second method I have used to enhance molecular Hydrogen in my drinking water is a Turapur[9] filter. I use a two-stage carbon filter to provide drinking water at my kitchen sink. I then fill a Turapur water filter[10] from that carbon-filtered water source. Thirdly, I fill a 16-17 ounce glass water bottle from the Turapur filter, which I drink out of personally. If I use an H2 tablet, I will let it dissolve within my glass bottle and drink it immediately. I can attest that the water from the Turapur water pitcher tastes better than the two-stage carbon-filtered water.

In summary, molecular hydrogen (H2) enhanced water can be essential in healing various diseases, especially[11] cancer.

Deuterium Depleted Water (DDW)

Virtually all sources of water contain some amount of deuterium[12]. The closer to the North and South poles or higher elevations, the less deuterium is found in the water. In contrast, the closer to the equator and lower elevations, the more deuterium is found in the water. See the noted internet reference for a complete discussion on this subject.

If you can understand deuterium-depleted water, it can help defeat your cancer and heal your body. If I found myself with cancer, I would consume deuterium-depleted water (DDW) as one of the healing protocols I would follow. This type of water can be purchased[13] (expensive) or created free (time-consuming) using a triple water freezing process[14].

Deuterium in higher concentrations can be destructive to biological processes. In lower concentrations, it can be healing to the body. Specifically, deuterium-depleted water consumption is believed to have the ability to flush[15] cancer out of the interstitium.

Deuterium is an isotope of Hydrogen that contains both a proton and a neutron in its nucleus, found in some Hydrogen molecules. A regular Hydrogen molecule has a single proton and no neutron. That makes a regular molecule of Hydrogen lighter than one with a deuterium isotope. Deuterium Hydrogen (see online reference studies[16]) can replace regular Hydrogen in water molecules, resulting in what is known as deuterium-enriched water. The deuterium concentration in water is typically expressed as parts per million (ppm).

"On the surface of the earth, there is about one deuterium atom in ocean water for every 6420 Hydrogen atoms. In other words, the deuterium concentration[17] for most of our planet's water is about 150-160 parts per million (ppm) or 0.000156%."

Deuterium levels in water can affect biological

systems, including the body's interstitium. The interstitium is the fluid-filled space between tissue cells, and it plays a crucial role in various physiological processes. Changes in deuterium levels can influence the composition and properties of this fluid, which in turn can impact cellular function.

Lower deuterium levels in water can lead to a reduction in interstitial deuterium concentration. That can affect the electrical properties of the interstitium, potentially altering the electrical potential across cell membranes and affecting cell communication and signaling. Lower deuterium levels have also been associated with improved mitochondrial function, as deuterium acts as a metabolic inhibitor.

On the other hand, higher water deuterium levels can increase deuterium concentration in the interstitium. This can disrupt the normal functioning of cellular processes, including energy production and various metabolic pathways. High deuterium levels are linked to oxidative stress, reduced cellular resilience, and increased risk of certain diseases.

Maintaining an optimal balance of deuterium levels in water is essential for maintaining cellular function and overall health. While some deuterium in water is natural and inevitable, excessive or imbalanced levels can harm the interstitium and various biological processes.

Potential Anti-cancer Effects

Some studies suggest that deuterium-depleted water may inhibit the growth of cancer cells. Deuterium might interfere with DNA replication, and reducing its water concentration could slow down cancer cell division.

Improved Athletic Performance

Some proponents claim that drinking deuterium-depleted water can enhance physical performance and recovery by improving mitochondrial function and reducing oxidative stress. Mitochondria are the energy-producing organelles in cells, and deuterium might affect their efficiency.

Anti-aging Effects

Deuterium-depleted water could have anti-aging properties by reducing oxidative damage to cells and tissues. Some animal studies have shown promising results regarding increased lifespan and improved health span. Still, more research is needed to determine if these effects translate to humans.

Improved Metabolic Health

There's some speculation that deuterium-depleted water might help regulate metabolism and improve insulin sensitivity, potentially offering benefits for weight management and diabetes prevention.

Enhanced Cognitive Function

Some proponents suggest that reducing deuterium levels in the body could improve cognitive function and protect against neurodegenerative diseases. See the notes for resources and study materials for deuterium-depleted water (DDW).

Body's Water Composition

I have already mentioned that our bodies are thought to comprise 60-75% water. That is a common belief and understanding. However, our body can also be viewed from a molecular weight perspective. In that case, our body is 98.9% water. We are, in essence, a water being from the viewpoint of our total molecular weight.

The Interstitium

The interstitium is a fluid-filled space in the body's connective tissues. It is a network of interconnected compartments lined by a layer of endothelial cells and supported by a matrix of collagen and other proteins.

Water plays a crucial role in the interstitium, helping maintain its structure and function. The fluid within the interstitium, known as interstitial fluid, is derived from plasma (the fluid part of the blood) and serves as a communication highway between cells and blood vessels. It transports nutrients, oxygen, and hormones to the cells while removing waste products and metabolic byproducts.

Various factors, including water intake and distribution in the body, regulate the amount and composition of interstitial fluid. When water intake is insufficient, dehydration can occur, leading to a decrease in interstitial fluid volume. That can have adverse effects on cell function and overall tissue health. On the other hand, excessive fluid intake or impaired fluid regulation mechanisms can cause fluid accumulation in the interstitium, leading to conditions such as edema characterized by swelling and tissue damage.

Water also influences the concentration of electrolytes, such as sodium and potassium, in the interstitium. Maintaining the balance of these electrolytes is crucial for cell function, nerve conduction, and fluid balance within the body.

Water is essential for the proper functioning of the interstitium. It influences the volume and composition of interstitial fluid, which plays a vital role in delivering nutrients and removing waste products from cells, maintaining tissue health, and regulating fluid balance in the body.

The Fascia

The fascia is a sheet of connective tissue that covers, supports, and separates the body's muscles, organs, and other structures. It is a protective layer that allows muscles, tendons, and other structures to move without friction or damage.

The fascia comprises collagen fibers and other proteins that give it strength and flexibility. It forms a continuous network throughout the body, connecting various parts and providing structural support and ease of movement for body parts.

Dehydration and a sedentary lifestyle will affect the ability to move different body parts. If you do not move the body regularly, the fascia around the muscles not being moved can dry up. That can result in the inability to move an arm, leg, or other body part that is not being used.

Grandma's adage of using or losing it is an absolute truism; our body's fascia is why. If you want to start using a wheelchair early in life, become a couch potato and don't move your body parts for extended periods. Again, not moving body parts causes certain parts of the fascia to dry up. If you are dehydrated at the same time the body is not moving, it can be dramatically worse. Yes, our bodies need water, and we need to move our body parts, or we could lose mobility in our legs, arms, hands, fingers, etc. Anecdotal thoughts from the past meet modern health sciences to explain what Grandma took for granted in days past.

Interstitium Vs. Fascia

While the interstitium and the fascia are types of connective tissue, they differ in their structures and functions. The fascia is a fibrous tissue that forms a sheath-like layer around muscles and separates different structures. At the same time, the interstitium primarily consists of fluid-filled spaces *between* cells where metabolic processes occur. The fascia mainly provides support and protection, while the interstitium plays a role in fluid balance, transport of nutrients, and immune response.

Water Is Healing!

Staying hydrated, consuming molecular Hydrogen (H2) enhanced water, and drinking deuterium-depleted water (DDW) improve the body's health. All three would be essential protocols for people with cancer, even if one had to produce deuterium-depleted water using the triple-freezing water protocol due to the high cost of purchasing this type of water.

CHAPTER TWELVE
Cancer 101

My Personal List

Considering some basic knowledge[1] about cancer, other diseases, and healing is appropriate. So, I've compiled a list of items I think are common sense do's and don'ts if I had a cancer diagnosis. Regardless of the disease, this list is a good one to review for any life-threatening disease, especially for cancer or other death diagnoses. This is neither a list of priorities nor a comprehensive list. Review the items on the list and determine if you need to think about or take action on any of them. A second list and comments follow. This list[2] is found in the book "*The Only Answer to Cancer*," Sixth Edition, © 2012, by Dr. Leonard Coldwell[3].

1. What is your relationship[4] with God?
2. You need to be proactive[5] with disease and healing
3. What is your purpose[6] for living? Why are you here?

4. You need to take responsibility for healing
5. Focus on treating your body, not the disease[7]
6. You need to believe in your body's ability to heal[8]
7. Do not fear cancer; over 300[9] alternative cures exist
8. You cannot rely on medical doctors to heal cancer
9. Standard medical practices do not heal cancer[10]
10. Focus on increasing the body's oxygen[11] levels
11. Avoid all processed meats
12. Avoid all processed foods
13. Avoid all vegetable seed oils[12]
14. Avoid white processed sugars
15. Avoid other sugar[13] products
16. Don't drink water out of plastic[14] bottles
17. Don't microwave cook in plastic containers
18. Don't store food in a plastic container
19. Do an elimination diet when allergies are present
20. Eliminate any food that offends the body
21. Do a spiritual[15] detox
22. Do an emotional or trauma[16] detox
23. Do an environmental[17] detox
24. Do a dental[18] fillings detox
25. Do a heavy metal detox for the body[19]
26. Do a parasitic detox
27. Systematically eliminate stress[20] in your life
28. Determine what works or makes you happy
29. Eliminate what doesn't work or stresses you

30. Eliminate toxic relationships that cause stress
31. Resolve *childhood* traumas[21]
32. Use Intermittent fasting to help the body heal
33. Use Time-Restricted eating as a way to fast
34. Skip the ketone[22] diets, your brain needs glucose
35. Eat only organic Whole Foods[23]
36. Eat organic raw foods when possible
37. Cook organic raw foods if needed
38. Make warm stews and soups if needed
39. Incorporate 30 minutes of sunlight daily
40. Supplement with Vitamin D3[24]
41. Vitamin D and A are symbiotic together.
42. Consider hyperthermia[25] protocols for healing
43. A simple shop halogen lamp can be hyperthermic
44. Consider methylene blue as a healing modality
45. Consider Chloride Dioxide (CDS) as a healing modality

Dr. Leonard Coldwell's List

Dr. Coldwell states: "What I've discovered, through the years, is that cancer is the easiest condition to cure! *In fact, there are over 300 proven ways to cure cancer naturally.* You can eliminate tumors and mutated cell growth with:

- Vitamin B17 (Laetrille)
- 35% food-grade hydrogen peroxide
- Vitamin C or Aloe Vera injections
- Essiac tea or capsules
- Turmeric
- Various mushrooms
- Oxygen or ozone therapy
- Vitamin D or sunlight
- Raw food or macrobiotic diets
- Full body and organ cleanse
- DMSO and Cesium chloride therapy
- Chinese Happy Tree
- Graviola fruit
- Triphala (Ayurvedic)
- Gerson therapy - a mixture of diet and supplementation
- Hemp or Hoxsey Therapy
- Enzyme therapy
- Hydrosol Silver
- Omega 3 fatty acids
- Eggplant (BEC-5)
- Baking soda and maple syrup
- Chelation therapy
- Photoluminescence
- Brussels sprouts, broccoli sprouts, garlic, green tea, spinach, or tomatoes

- Echinacea
- Folic acid
- Lacto-Terrine enzymes
- Saw palmetto
- Selenium
- Minerals

Many other herbs, foods, and supplements can cure the symptoms of what they call cancer."

Warning: *If you are diagnosed with cancer, medical doctors will put extreme pressure on you to take immediate action.[26] They may even schedule surgery, radiation, or chemo within a few days of your cancer diagnosis without your consent. Do not succumb to the fears of dying without immediate standard-of-care medical procedures. It took years for your body to get to this point. Your body will wait some more time to get fully informed of your treatment options by reading Dr. Leonard Coldwell's book: "The Only Answer To Cancer." The statistical reality is that only 2-3% of people ever survive standard medical treatment procedures for cancers. Ask the doctor pressuring you how long they will guarantee you will live if you agree to their rushed treatment procedures. Their answer might surprise you.*

CHAPTER THIRTEEN
Nutrition & Cancer

**"<u>Understanding</u> is a *wellspring of life* to
him [or her] who has it." Proverbs 16:22**

The Bible states that people can die for lack of
instruction, knowledge, and understanding. In contrast,
understanding is said to be a wellspring (continual
source) of life to those who possess it. So, let's discuss
other issues concerning healing and the impact of
nutrients at the cellular level. I hope that your
understanding of healing and what your body is up
against with cancer will increase.

God has placed tremendous healing power at the
cellular level inside our body. Each cell is akin to a small
manufacturing plant. Like the electricity and utilities that
keep our homes functioning, our cells require various
nutrients to function correctly. It is a fact that the body
wants to heal itself if supplied with the nutrition it needs
to heal. Like a car that needs fuel, our bodies run on the
nutrition we provide.

Billions of cells die each day we live, and new ones are created. This cycle of cellular death and life in our bodies keeps us alive. However, sickness and disease occur if something goes awry at the cellular level. Nutrition can make our body friendly to disease or highly resistant to disease.

Some time ago, I caught a television special on alternative nutrition. One example on the show was a man who had pancreatic cancer and was sent home to die. As he and his wife searched for an alternative healing option, they wound up in the New York City office of an alternative doctor. These are doctors who use nutraceutical products instead of or in addition to pharmaceutical products. Let me explain.

When I talk about nutrition in the cellular sense, I am talking about the food found in vitamins, herbs, greens, and other supplements. Of course, natural food sources such as vegetables and fruits are also important from a cellular point of view, as are limited amounts of proteins and fats. However, instead of pushing pharmaceutical drugs, alternative medical doctors specialize in treating the body's needs at a cellular level with natural nutrients, including what types of healing foods to eat. Their healing concept is simple: feed the body what it needs from a nutritional perspective, and the body can then heal itself.

When finished, the pancreatic cancer patient left the doctor's office with instructions to consume about 100 nutraceutical pills per day. He was also told to take four coffee enemas daily to clean out his colon. Strangely enough, in 2003, my early cancer research came to similar conclusions for the pancreatic cancer my first wife was stricken with. She ruled out coffee enemas. I also had to restrict her pill intake to 50 per day at a maximum.

For anyone who has never consumed a lot of vitamins, 50 pills/day is a mountain to climb. God has given me a couple of insights about this. First, pray for yourself while you are healthy because when you are sick and on a deathbed, you may have to rely on others. It may be difficult during those times when you are ill or on a deathbed. Secondly, when seriously sick, consuming any food, let alone a volume of pills, is often challenging. Especially 50-100 per day!

My first wife couldn't deal with the volume of nutrients needed daily to fight the cancer. The man traveling to New York died after five months. I suspect he also couldn't take in the volume of nutrients needed. I was sick once, for a couple of weeks, and I can tell you that I couldn't take in the nutraceuticals [pills] I usually consumed. Typically, this would be close to 50 pills in the morning and at least another 20 or more in the evening.

Therefore, one major problem when stage IV cancer

sets in is the sheer volume of nutrients that are needed to counteract the onslaught of the cancer at the body's cellular level. When we are healthy, it is difficult to maintain the discipline to consume a large amount of nutraceutical pills. When we are sick or on a deathbed with this requirement being a necessity, it is a good bet that some help from the family will be needed to allow such an intake of nutrients and keep you on schedule.

Today, there is an attack from pharmaceutical companies and various government agencies (shills) against alternative medical technologies and most nutritional supplements (nutraceuticals). I know of one person thrown into jail for selling apricot seeds and the drug form of its vitamin B17 (laetrile), a little-known cancer-fighting nutrient. I know of two alternative medicine doctors that the FDA raided and tried to shut down because of their cancer-fighting practices. Alternative doctor offices have also been raided for selling nutraceuticals like Vitamins, Minerals, etc.

It is a sad commentary that if you want the best alternative healing treatments for fighting cancer, you may have to go to Mexico or another country. If the pharmaceutical companies have their way, you might need a prescription to purchase any vitamins, minerals, or other nutraceuticals that are currently available over the counter. Efforts are also being made to limit the quantity of Vitamin C and other nutrients to such low values that they would be useless from a healing perspective. There is such a concept as the therapeutic dosage of nutraceuticals like Vitamin C, etc. For example, therapeutic doses range from 25,000 to 100,000 mg for fighting cancer using Vitamin C, administered via an IV whenever possible. It is the easiest way to get that amount of Vitamin C into the body.

Don't think for a moment that I am joking. I am not. Nutrient knowledge, which is very limited in the public's know-how, is being threatened with extinction through powerful and evil forces. It is Satan at work in the realm of our ability to heal our bodies nutritionally. The first time you hear about laws affecting vitamins and other nutraceuticals, contact your politicians and tell them not to mess with their widespread availability. Tell them to restrict all regulatory agencies from limiting the availability of any nutrient or nutraceutical.

Laws already passed in Europe make therapeutic doses of some vitamins and minerals available only with a doctor's prescription. Drugs are dumped on society with as little as 3,000 human trials. When the drug kills people, no one finds out until a drug company insider blows the whistle or an injured person's lawsuit is found successful in a Court. Why are nutritional products used by millions of people, like vitamins and minerals, being threatened?

Warning: Keep a watchful eye out. Why are nutraceuticals like vitamins and minerals needed? They are necessary because the nutrients we used to get in foods have been depleted and stripped away. It is the direct result of topsoil erosion, genetically modified foods (GMOs), chemical fertilizers, and pre-shelf food treatments such as irradiation that kill off the natural enzymes everyday foods possess. You might have already experienced the joys of GMO foods, like a beautiful tomato with no taste compared to one grown out of a local garden or from an organic farmer.

12 Healing Facts

1. Our bodies need enzymes for various cellular tasks. They have been stripped out of our food sources. While our bodies create enzymes, as much as 50% of what our bodies need is no longer available from the foods that we eat. Supplemental enzyme products are now available to offset this reality. A lack of enzymes might be responsible for or significant in many modern sicknesses and diseases. Purchase organic foods to get foods with enzymes.

2. Some nutraceuticals are now available in liquid form, which allows us to consume therapeutic amounts

and reduce the volume of "pill intake." A liquid form is particularly helpful when the quantity of pills is too high and can be more easily consumed. Vitamin C is also available in liquid form or can be created in liquid form from powder. This is useful when Vitamin C--IV treatment is not locally available.

3.   Empty gel capsules in various sizes can be obtained online[1]. Nutrients can be ground up and then stuffed in the gel capsules for easier intake. These gel capsules can also be filled with the powdered form of various nutrients, which are often less expensive.

4.   Gel capsules can be taken via the anus and rectally if they cannot be tolerated through the stomach.

5.   Medicines can also be placed inside larger gel capsules and then taken via the anus if they cannot be taken orally or tolerated in the stomach.

6.   A properly functioning body can have a bowel movement after almost every meal.

7.   When the colon is cleansed, it can eliminate 7-21 pounds of waste material stuck to its sides. A clean colon allows the body to dispose of waste and toxins more efficiently.

8.   Disease can flourish on the inside walls of our large intestine and colon. Regularly cleaning the body's colon minimizes this disease-breeding zone. It is equally essential to ensure the anus is kept clean after bowel

movements[2].

9. Just eating fruit seeds can be a cure for cancer. Most fruit seeds contain vitamin B17, and all fruit seeds have the same bitter cherry-like taste. Bite into apple seeds that you eat so the vitamin B17 is absorbed in your body. In other words, eat the whole apple.

10. The Internet is a knowledge base for communications and research. As a result, many cancer cures are being documented on alternative health websites.

11. A pH test of your saliva can tell whether or not your body is friendly or resistant to disease. Your body should test alkaline with a pH of 7 or more. A healthy body can measure 7.4. An alkaline pH reading means the body is resistant to disease. An acidic pH test means the body is more friendly to disease.

12. L-lysine and Vitamin C, in combination in large volumes, can prevent cancer from spreading by strengthening the collagen fibers. That can help with stage IV cancers when metastasis has occurred. Alternatively, collagen products are readily available to purchase online[3].

Most medical doctors remain uninformed on therapeutic nutrient and nutraceutical approaches to treating cancer. Cancer treatment is big business in the

United States. It is a 150-billion-dollar industry[4]. Do you think the industry wants you to eat fruit seeds and consume inexpensive nutrients or nutraceuticals to heal your body? Absolutely not. Their best business strategy is to stifle alternative nutraceutical healing information availability[5]. They often use the government as an enforcer to limit the introduction of alternative nutrients or nutritional cancer cures.

Apricots and other fruit seeds[6], like Apple seeds and their chemical equivalent, laetrile, are sources of vitamin B17. These are natural to the human body, and we used to get B17 nutrition in the fruit seeds that were crushed and mixed into jams and jellies, etc. Cultures and societies exist in the world where cancer is unheard of, and vitamin B17 consumption is one reason.

When I started eating apricot seeds[7], a rich source of B17, I noticed a black growth on my right leg that shrunk and fell off. Some of my friends had a similar experience at the same time with unwanted growths on their bodies. One seed per day per 10 pounds of body weight was considered safe to consume daily, and up to six seeds in a given hour. When my dying wife and I reached 15 seeds a day, both of our blood pressures dropped by 25 points. Unbelievable. I also had another growth on my shoulder, which shrank and disappeared. My wife had wanted me to see a doctor about it. Apricot seeds and laetrile were our number one weapon to fight the cancer in my wife's body. A good multivitamin and mineral package with greens is also helpful to allow the body to heal.

L-lysine and Vitamin C in high volumes minimize the spread of cancer. Daily therapeutic doses of 12,000 to 25,000 mg of each nutrient are suggested to prevent cancer from metastasizing to other body locations. I found a source of liquid Vitamin C[8] that proved helpful in reducing the volume of pills I needed. I also located liquid vitamins A and E that allowed therapeutic doses of those nutrients.

I found many other nutraceuticals, like liquid oxygen. Cancer cells do not like an oxygenated body or high temperatures. Enhancing the intake of oxygen can destroy cancer cells. Applying heat locally near tumors can raise their temperature and kill cancer cells.

One of my more exciting discoveries was the Budwig diet designed by Dr. Johanna Budwig. The combination of organic cottage cheese and flaxseed oil was shown to be a powerful cure for cancer by oxygenating the body and supplying it with abundant free electrons. Budwig's recipe is to consume three tablespoons of flaxseed oil mixed with eight ounces of organic 1-2% cottage cheese daily. I am sure you get the picture. There are many nutraceutical and food approaches to killing cancer.

When your loved one receives a death diagnosis from

an allopathic doctor, why should it matter to the Medical Industry what you do in terms of seeking a cure? It shouldn't. However, if the public suddenly learned how to keep their bodies healthy and, via DIY self-care healing strategies, eliminate or even cure disease, powerful drug companies and the Medical Industry would lose a lot of business. You might be surprised that you don't even crave junk food when your body is healthy at the cellular level. In other words, a healthy body has fewer bad habits. Of course, this is another chicken-and-egg scenario for you to think through.

Cancer thrives on sugars, junk food, and processed food because those foods feed a fermentation growth process. Deny the body access to the nutrients that cancer wants and supply it with the nutrients your cells need to fight cancer. Healing is then generated at the cellular level. This was God's plan when HE taught us in Genesis what we should eat as our food.

"And God said, 'See, I have given you every herb that yields seed which is on the face of all the earth, and every tree whose fruit yields seed; to you it shall be for food.' " Genesis 1:29

Catch the part about seeds. My wife might have been

naturally healed by food from her garden had it been planted the previous year before she died. Her source of the body nutrients she needed came from the garden she tended each year. Mine came from nutraceutical products. I took the position that I usually ate junk food and needed nutraceuticals. She took the position that she usually ate good food. Ultimately, ongoing cellular health is achieved by giving the body God gave us the nutrition its cells need. If you need healing, you should also stop eating processed food. It would help if you also stopped consuming or cooking with modern seed oils like corn oil, etc.

If God didn't make it, don't eat it! Nutritionally speaking, that simple advice is the best food advice any cancer patient will ever receive. I'm sure that many doctors might disagree. I know of one cancer patient who was told to consume sugar by his doctor. Yikes!

I studied cancer for three weeks full-time before my first wife died in 2003. I've now studied cancer for over 20 years. I am amazed by the many alternative nutraceutical healing strategies that exist and are suppressed by the medical industry and their government collaborators.[9] It isn't just cancer-cure information that is censored; many other diseases also suffer from censorship.

You can't count on the American Cancer Association (ACA) and other non-profit organizations like it. They are not in the business of teaching you about low-cost disease cures. They are tied to the Medical Industry, Big Pharma, and its significant annual revenues from treating the disease they claim to want to cure. However, they only desire to provide comfort and assurance that someone is trying to find a cure for whatever disease the organization represents. It is one reason I have started two health blogs[10] on my author's website[11].

Don't wait until you are confronted with stage III or stage IV metastasized cancer in your body to change your habits. Start your healing today by changing your lifestyle and adopting better health habits before you get sick. God said we could live to 120 years[12] of age. HE also said we could have a life with a future and hope[13]. Yet, you are in the driver's seat regarding your health and longevity. If you want the best of God's Grace and Mercy, give HIM your best health habits.

It is mythology that prayer will always bring healing. Prayer is essential to healing, but it cannot be the only part. The Word of God has many attributes of healing. HIS sovereignty, GRACE, and MERCY all play a role.

Solomon Taught

"*Have two goals:* wisdom--that is, knowing and doing right--and common sense. Don't let them slip away, for they fill you with living energy and bring you honor and respect. They keep you safe from defeat and disaster and from stumbling off the trail. With them on guard you can sleep without fear; you need not be afraid of disaster or the plots of wicked men, for the LORD is with you; he protects you." Proverbs 3:21-24 LIV

"*Wisdom Gives*: A Long, Good Life; Riches; Honor; Pleasure; and, Peace." Proverbs 3:16-17 LIV

When you submit your life and will to God, HE will take care of you in ways you cannot imagine. That includes the gift of healing and also the gift of eternal life in a heavenly mansion.

CHAPTER FOURTEEN
Sugar & Cancer

Sugar is the main ingredient that cancer feeds on. It's almost axiomatic that if a loved one is bedridden and dying of cancer, some family member will bring out a box of chocolate candies when they come to visit. Yes, it is a gift of love. However, it also exemplifies just how ignorant we are collectively about cancer and what cancer feeds on. Otherwise, good-intentioned loved ones would not show up with candies that might expedite the death of their sick family member whom they came to visit, maybe to say a final goodbye.

According to one doctor[1] whose newsletter I subscribed to, if you want to eliminate your cancer risk, eliminate sugar in your diet. Supposing you wanted to eliminate sugar from your diet, good luck, as sugar is now added to thousands of food products most of us consume to enhance the taste, like ketchup, canned fruit, bread, etc. Everyone knows that our bodies derive energy from sugar, aka glucose.

The modern Keto diet craze seeks to take advantage

of the fact that if we starve our bodies of sugar and other glucose products, our bodies will burn fat cells for energy. However, it has become more complicated than skipping glucose and burning fat. In the long run, a Keto diet could pose other health problems. Why? Our brains prefer to burn glucose instead of fats for energy, even though the brain can survive fat-burning for a while.

If you're thinking about going on a Keto diet to lose weight, research what is emerging as possible adverse effects. I need to learn more about Keto before commenting further on this issue.

I don't worry about the natural sugars found in fruits. However, I avoid all processed foods, which can be loaded with sugars and other undesirable ingredients. I try to avoid all foods using processed white sugar. I avoid high fructose corn syrup (HFCS) whenever possible, as it is unnatural to the human body. There is mounting evidence that HFCS[2] may be an underlying cause of obesity in America.

"Fructose goes straight to your liver and starts a fat production factory," Dr. Hyman says. "It triggers the production of triglycerides and cholesterol." (See noted HFCS article.)

CHAPTER FIFTEEN
Food & Cancer

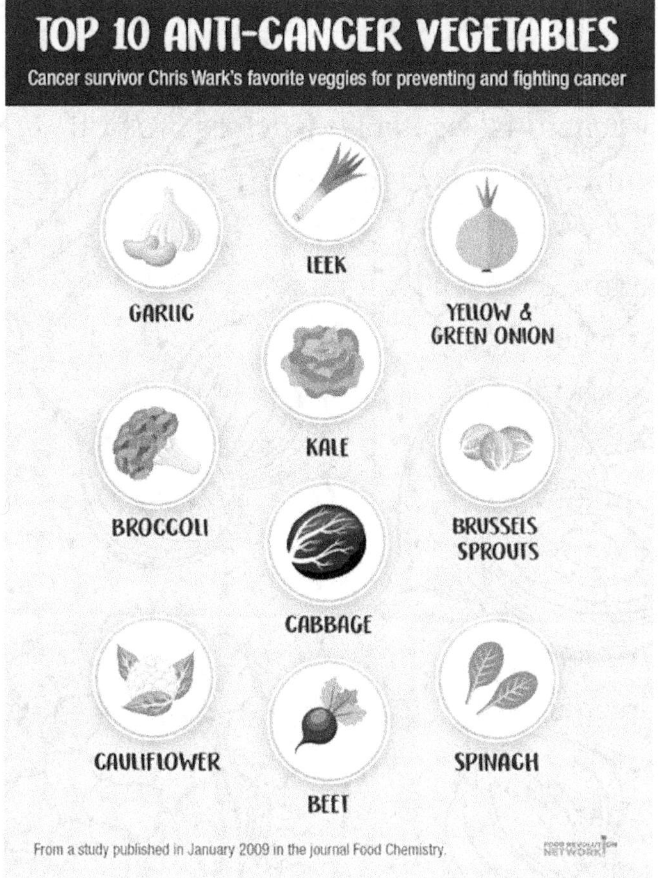

The ***Food***[1] ***Revolution Network*** is your best resource[2] for natural and healing food advice.

Cancer Fighting Foods List[3]

1) Berries (such as blueberries, blackberries, raspberries, and strawberries)
2) Green leafy vegetables (such as spinach, kale, and collard greens)
3) Cruciferous vegetables (such as broccoli, cauliflower, cabbage, and Brussels sprouts)
4) Leeks
5) Yellow & Green Onions
6) Artichokes
7) Avocados
8) Beets
9) Cinnamon
10) Tomatoes
11) Garlic
12) Turmeric
13) Green tea
14) Apples
15) Flaxseeds
16) Lemons
17) Olive Oil
18) Dark Chocolate

     God And Cancer: A Self-Care Perspective

19) Pomegranates

20) Ginger

21) Walnuts

22) Other nuts

23) Green Tea

24) Ginseng

25) Mushrooms

Food categories that increase cancer:

1) **Processed meats:** Studies have shown that consuming processed meats like hot dogs, bacon, and deli meats may be linked to an increased risk of certain types of cancer, particularly colorectal cancer.

2) **Red meat:** High consumption of red meat, especially when grilled or charred at high temperatures, has been associated with a higher risk of colorectal cancer and other types of cancer.

3) **Ultra-processed[4] foods are linked to 32 Illnesses:** Early death, heart disease, cancer, mental health disorders, overweight and obesity, and type 2 diabetes. This category would include packaged snacks, sugary drinks, instant noodles, sweet cereals, and ready-to-eat meals.

4) **Sugary drinks:** High intake of sugary beverages has been linked to an increased risk of obesity and certain types of cancers, such as pancreatic cancer.

5) **Trans fats:** Foods high in trans fats, such as commercially baked goods, fried foods, and processed snacks, may increase the risk of certain cancers.

Dangerous Seed Oils To Avoid

1) Sunflower seed oil
2) Canola oil
3) Corn oil
4) Soybean oil
5) Safflower oil
6) Cottonseed oil
7) Sesame oil
8) Peanut oil

The above seed oils contain high levels of linoleic acid (LA). While famous for cooking, these seed oils can cause dangerous inflammation within the body. Avoid these seed oils to improve your health if you fight cancer or other health issues. Linoleic acid is an omega-6 fatty acid commonly found in vegetable oils.

However, other cooking oils, such as olive, avocado,

and coconut, do not contain high levels of linoleic acid. These oils contain different fatty acid profiles and may better suit health needs.

The health issue involved is an overabundance of omega-6 fatty acids in our modern diets and insufficient omega-3 fatty acids. In alternative health circles, using the vegetable seed oils in the above "avoid list" is often considered an underlying cause of most chronic health conditions.

It's recommended to focus on using olive and avocado oils for cooking.

According to alternative Doctor Al Sears, cruciferous[5] vegetables are essential to winning your personal war on cancer because they contain sulforaphane. Dr. Sears explains why in his new book[6]. He also identifies other cancer healing protocols.

"Sulforaphane neutralizes toxins, calms inflammation, and puts the brakes on tumor growth. In fact, one study found that just eating three to five servings of cruciferous vegetables a week cuts your risk of cancer by 40%."

<u>Troublesome Grains To Avoid</u>

Gluten has become an issue with **wheat, barley, oats, and rye** grains. These grain products are now associated with various illnesses and even cancer in America. It is also reported that people affected in the USA may not have a problem with these grains when they travel to Europe. It has been reported that this is because glyphosate (Roundup) is used on grain crops at harvest time in the USA to dry the crops. If you have a severe illness, like cancer, your best strategy would be to avoid all of these grains to eliminate their influence on your healing.

CHAPTER SIXTEEN
Exercise & Cancer

I used to be a runner and go to the gym for an hour of exercise five days a week. I stopped running at 13.5 miles due to tendinitis in the right shoulder. Unfortunately, I never got started running again. I stopped the gym routine when I moved. I also invested an estimated $15-20k into my own gym. At one point, I was enamored with exercise and its accompanying machines and devices to improve my body.

In the 70s, running was all the rage from an exercise perspective. It was designed to improve our heart's aerobic capacity. However, a well-known aerobic running guru[1] who authored *"The Complete Book On Running"* died while jogging at age 52 from a heart attack. Focusing on aerobic endurance running was an unwise exercise strategy for the heart. The problem turns out to be conditioning the heart in a way that doesn't factor in the body's "fight or flight" response system. In other words, endurance running might make it incapable of reacting with the proper physiological response when we need our hearts to kick into gear.

The issue with the '70s aerobic conditioning strategy of endurance running is that it can place too much emphasis on long-duration, low-intensity aerobic exercise without adequate heart variation or intensity. While endurance running can benefit cardiovascular health, exclusively relying on this exercise is not optimal for overall heart health.

Studies have shown that high-intensity interval training (HIIT) and strength training can also play important roles in heart health by improving cardiovascular fitness, increasing heart strength, and promoting better cardiac function. In addition to heart training issues, continuous endurance running can lead to overuse injuries, muscle imbalances, and excessive wear and tear on the body.

I eventually decided that the need for any form of exercise that required a machine or going to a gym was not what I needed. I am convinced that moderately moving the body is what our human body needs. However, our modern lifestyles involve too much sitting, which is dangerous to our health.

According to Dr. Joseph Mercola[2], we should limit sitting to three hours or less (a day) and avoid sitting for more than 50 minutes at a time. Good luck with that recommendation. I'm trying, but I am not there, at least not yet. I do a lot of computer work during the day. That has led me to purchase a standing desk, which I can lower or raise as needed. I do most of my writing sitting in a massage chair. Often, I get into a state of flow where hours can pass unnoticed. So, I must be more mindful to ensure I am moving my body more often.

The body's movement in moderation interests me the most in my life. Sitting can sometimes cause my lower back pain. As little as 5 minutes of Yoga stretches can eliminate the pain. In the Mercola article, he lists the following seven realities about our bodies.

1. Prolonged sitting takes a toll even if you exercise.
2. Exercise cannot undo the damage of prolonged sitting.
3. Excessive sitting is the riskiest for women.
4. Excessive sitting leads to exhausted workers.
5. Moderate physical activity cannot be overdone.
6. Too much vigorous exercise backfires.
7. Overdoing strength training is worse than doing none.

Why does a sedentary lifestyle cause so much harm?

"Muscular[3] and cellular systems that process blood sugar, triglycerides, and cholesterol are activated simply by carrying your bodyweight upon your legs."

It is the regular movement of our body that will keep us healthy. However, exercise can be overdone, and I know of three people who have injured themselves from aggressive exercising. Dr. Mercola is an avid exerciser and is deeply involved in studying the impact of exercise on the human body.

What amount of maximum exercise does Dr. Mercola think is helpful to strive for in a given week?

Dr. Mercola's Exercise Program

1) 40-60 minutes max of strength[4] training.
2) 75 minutes max of high-intensity[5] training.
3) Walking[6] as much as possible during the day.

As an active senior, I have noticed many seniors seeking to ease their lives by obtaining an electric wheelchair. Many shoppers of various ages at the local grocery store use sit-down shopping carts. Disabled people need to use the electric chairs, however, I have noticed many able-bodied people using them. Without realizing it, they are harming their bodies and would do better walking.

Warning: If you can walk, even if it's difficult or you need a cane, it's better to do so for as long as possible. This also means that if you can tolerate some pain while walking, walking is better than riding in an electric wheelchair. Sitting when you can stand or walk only harms your health.

I used to be a runner many decades ago. When I first attempted to run, I ran out of breath, somewhere between 50 and 100 feet from where I started. At that point, I walked to regain my breath. This brings up a discussion about high-intensity interval training (HIIT). Dr. Al Sears has an exercise program called PACE[7]. I first read about this exercise program over 15 years ago. His website describes this HIIT program as follows:

Dr. Sears' PACE program

"If you want to get a taste for PACE[8], here are a few things you can do right now:

Find an exertion level: Push yourself until you are breathing heavily and until you feel it would be hard to carry on a conversation. You can do this by running, biking, riding a machine at the gym, etc.

Dynamic Rest:

1. Stop and recover.

2. Measure your heart rate. You can do that with a heart rate monitor or find your pulse.

3. Count the beats for six seconds and multiply by ten when you feel your heart beating. That's your pulse rate.

Record your progress: How long did it take you to reach a high level of exertion? How long did it take you to recover? What was your heart rate? Write it down."

As referenced in the notes, you can obtain Dr. Sears' PACE[9] program's full details on his website. When I first learned of the program, it was described as a 12-minute exercise program. A person would run until they were out of breath, walk until their breathing recovered, and repeat this run-walk HIIT sequence for twelve minutes. This cycle is a good way of obtaining aerobic exercise results without getting aggressive and injuring yourself.

From a movement perspective, it takes a limited amount of time to keep your body healthy each week between Dr. Mercola's and Dr. Sears's recommendations. It only takes prioritizing, willpower, and scheduling the time on your weekly calendar to make it happen. Failure to keep moving your body is equivalent to putting one foot into the grave. Regardless of age, especially if you are gravely ill, it is essential to keep moving.

Moving The Body
Is An Anti-Cancer Strategy

CHAPTER SEVENTEEN
Teeth & Cancer

When it comes to overall health, the condition of our teeth can have an enormous negative impact. It starts slowly with amalgam (mercury-based) fillings. As we age, it expands with crowns, root canals, gums, and other issues like teeth pulling and bridges.

I'll use my teeth as an example of what can go wrong. Just two years ago, at age 76, I experienced a stroke resulting from high blood pressure. For several months, I couldn't move my left eye to the left and, in the process, experienced double vision. The cause? It was a root canal that was eating away the bone in my upper jaw. So how did my body get there, and how did I get healed?

I often wondered if my family didn't inherit some tooth decay issue. I've noticed that some kids and grandkids have experienced enamel and other tooth decay issues. For me, it started when I was very young. I remember that, around the age of 12, I had to have significant fillings done on my front teeth and others. The dentist drilled holes into my front four teeth to remove the decay and then filled them in the best he could to match the color of the teeth. Of course, the side teeth were repaired and then filled with amalgam (mercury-based) filling. This was around 1958 in North Minneapolis.

I will take full blame for not brushing my teeth faithfully when I was young. However, I can't say how all this damage to my teeth materialized. I remember visiting the local bakery at 5 am as a paperboy and getting some excellent glazed donuts. They certainly could have been part of it.

I joined the Navy in August 1963 and left in December 1970. During that time, naval dentists diligently worked on my teeth. I remember several times when Navy dentists rebuilt my teeth from the gum line upwards using amalgam fillings. I'm always thankful for those dentists who resisted the urge to pull a tooth. Instead, I suspect they enjoyed the creativity of building a new tooth from one down to the gums or from almost scratch in the dentist's eyes.

Later in life, as additional work must be done, the dentist must drill deeper into the tooth. Eventually, the filling sits on the nerve (tooth's roots). Today, the dentist can place an isolation blanket over the nerve. Hence, the metal filling does not directly contact the tooth's roots.

Problems with teeth repair compound as a person

ages. Metal fillings eventually will result in tooth pain, resulting in a root canal procedure. This is where the tooth is drilled down into the roots, and they are extracted. The tooth roots are then filled with a solid material. Now, you have basically a dead tooth. If the tooth is still strong, you may get by for several years without issues. If the tooth is weak, the doctor will need to put a porcelain cap on top of the tooth.

My first root canal was done in my upper jaw about 24 years ago. It was cuspid #6 on the right, shown in the chart below. I immediately noticed gum tenderness when I pressed it near the tooth. Root canal teeth can get infected, resulting in an abscess that can swell up like a balloon and be painful. I eventually returned to the root canal dentist and said I thought something was wrong with the tooth. He did some testing and assured me it was okay.

In hindsight, the tooth was not okay. I now realize that I had a low-grade infection at the root of the tooth. I was also fortunate that the tooth had a natural drainage path from the root. I never experienced a nasty abscess or swelling of the gum and face resulting from this low-grade bacterial infection. I also realize dentists can never remove all the bacteria from a root canal procedure. This means that all root canals have bacterial infections that can flare up.

In my case, 22 years after the root canal procedure, that bacterial infection was eating my jawbone.

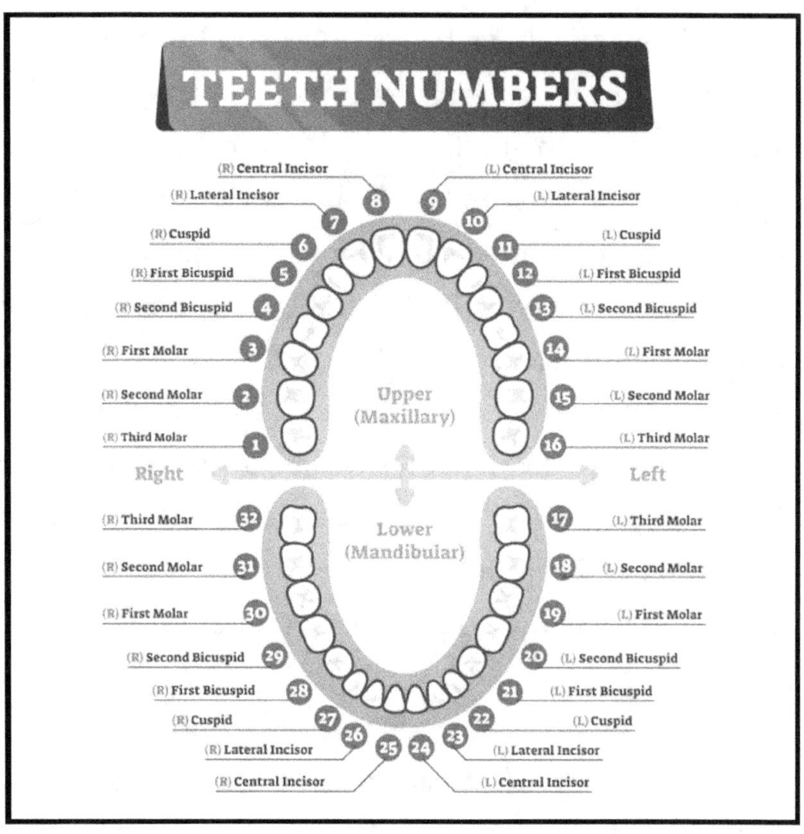

The blood that supplies the roots of all our teeth is tied directly to organs in the body. Remember, teeth are living organisms in our mouths. Teeth roots supply blood to the tooth to keep it alive. Once the tooth roots are removed, the tooth dies. The chart below illustrates which teeth are connected to which organs.

The fastest way to a heart attack would be ignoring your teeth when periodontal disease is present.

Tooth / Organ Relationship Chart

Right Side | Left Side

Upper (teeth 1–16)

Teeth	1	2	3	4	5	6	7	8	9	10	11	12	13	14	15	16
Upper Jaw	3rd Molar (wisdom)	2nd Molar	1st Molar	2nd Bicuspid (pre-molar)	1st Bicuspid (pre-molar)	Canine (cuspid)	lateral incisor	Central incisor	Central incisor	lateral incisor	Canine (cuspid)	1st Bicuspid (pre-molar)	2nd Bicuspid (pre-molar)	1st Molar	2nd Molar	3rd Molar (wisdom)

Lower (teeth 32–17)

Teeth	32	31	30	29	28	27	26	25	24	23	22	21	20	19	18	17
Lower Jaw	3rd Molar (wisdom)	2nd Molar	1st Molar	2nd Bicuspid (pre-molar)	1st Bicuspid (pre-molar)	Canine (cuspid)	lateral incisor	Central incisor	Central incisor	lateral incisor	Canine (cuspid)	1st Bicuspid (pre-molar)	2nd Bicuspid (pre-molar)	1st Molar	2nd Molar	3rd Molar (wisdom)

Element	Fire	Earth	Metal	Wood	Water	Water	Wood	Metal	Earth	Fire

In one study of breast cancers in women, 90% of the women had a root canal on the same side of their mouths as the cancerous breast. The reality of root canals has not caught up with most dentists. However, why should you leave a dead organ inside your body? A YouTube documentary, "Root Cause," explains how dangerous root canals can be to your health. You can find it at https://www.youtube.com/watch?v=OHN-JJO7HHw.

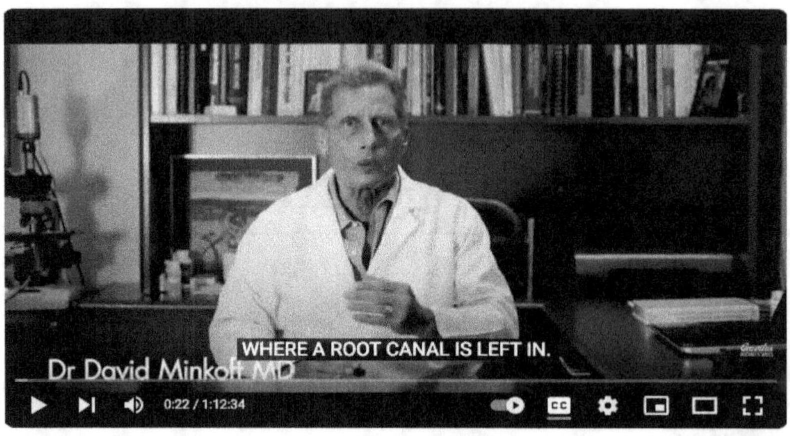

It took 22 years before the root canal infection grew to the point where the bacteria was literally eating away my upper jawbone. I didn't realize it was also at the point where my blood pressure had exploded past 190 systolic. I had been to the dentist and knew of the root canal issue. I decided to try some natural antibiotics and emphasize garlic. However, I was unaware that the infection was increasing my blood pressure.

My wife and I were going to a park in South Minneapolis. I was driving when I suddenly got exhausted and started seeing double of everything. I had suffered a stroke that affected the nerve that fed the muscle of my left eye, allowing the eye to move to the left. You can read about the incident and how I was healed in my book[1] "*The Doctor's Death Diagnosis.*"

Take care of your teeth to maintain a healthy body.

Request composite fillings to avoid metal fillings. Get all the metal in your teeth removed when you can afford it. Do not accept root canal procedures. Instead, have the tooth pulled. Have a non-metallic dental implant[2] procedure if you don't want to live with a missing tooth.

Teeth Affect The Body's Health
And Can Cause Cancer

CHAPTER EIGHTEEN
Sleep & Cancer

"You will keep him [or her] in perfect peace, whose mind is stayed on You, because he [or she] trusts in You." Isaiah 26:3

Sleep as a curative strategy for cancer is not something to be taken for granted. Sleep goes beyond being essential and becomes fundamental to healing for any severe disease. Why is that? It involves the distinction between our body's sympathetic nervous system and its parasympathetic nervous system.

Our bodies operate between two primary strategies. The first is sympathetic and represents when our bodies are in a "Fight or Flight" mode. The second is when our bodies are in a "Rest and Repair" mode, the parasympathetic.

The body cannot fully heal if it always operates in the sympathetic nervous system and never rests. This means, of course, you have to de-stress your life. It doesn't mean that you never experience stress. That would be impossible, and stress is required for the body to function normally. However, it means that you have to resolve any significant stress that creates anxiety and keeps you awake at night, unable to sleep.

<u>Sleep is when the body repairs itself!</u>

I plan for nine hours in bed to get eight hours of sleep. It's not always possible, but that is my primary sleep strategy. When I was a young man in my 20s and 30s, I didn't make provision for much sleep. In those days, if I got five hours, it was sufficient since I was otherwise working on my goals in life. However, on more than one occasion, when I pushed myself for 3-4 weeks on limited sleep, I managed to dent my car with insufficient mental clarity to see a concrete obstacle in a parking lot.

I've struggled with various obstacles to sleep. You may have one or more of these same issues preventing a sound sleep. Here are solutions that I've found effective.

If you are in pain, you can try nutraceutical solutions to see if they will help. 307mg of Boswellia[1] (Frankincense). I tested this version of Frankincense against 220mg of Naproxen (Aleve) and found it to be as effective. However, it is a natural ingredient, not a pharmaceutical drug. Pain is often directly related to deficiencies in the body's nutrients, especially in omega-3 fatty acids. My nutraceutical approach to getting rid of body pain is to use two of each of the following quantities of three nutraceuticals once or twice during the day. See notes for source.

1) 2 - Mega EFA[2] (Essential Fatty Acids)
2) 2 - Borage Oil[3] (Gamma Linoleic Acid)
3) 2 - Bromelain[4] (Pineapple Enzyme)

All three of these ingredients are low-cost solutions that eliminate pain in the body. They are also known to relieve pain associated with arthritis conditions. It is difficult to sleep if the body is in pain. You can also use a widely available microwave hot pack for muscle pain.

If your mind doesn't stop thinking, try the following nutraceuticals to slow it down and help you fall asleep.

1) GABA[5] (Gamma-Aminobutyric Acid)
2) L-Theanine[6]
3) Melatonin (1 mg)[7]

All three of these ingredients are highly effective at helping me sleep. A particular caution on Melatonin for sleep. Very high doses of melatonin are used to fight cancer. However, for sleep, it can be self-defeating. A 1mg dose was highly recommended by anti-aging Doctor Al Sears[8]. I've found his 1mg dosage advice accurate and had previously tried dosages of 3-12 mg to try to sleep. Suppose you are going to use Melatonin in high doses to fight cancer. In that case, you must work with an alternative doctor or naturopath.

If anxiety is keeping you awake, you can try Kava Kava. I'm talking about the anxiety that feels like a weight on your chest. When my first wife was diagnosed with terminal cancer, it felt like an elephant or a truck was on my chest, and I could barely breathe. I suspect my heart was also racing at the time. I already knew about Kava Kava[9]. 2,000 mg is what finally calmed my anxiety over the pending loss of my loved one. Kava is available in 234-500 mg capsules. I would recommend taking 1-2 if you are experiencing anxiety at this level. Kava is reported to conflict with alcohol and should not be taken if you are drinking alcohol of any type. In the past, I purchased Kava from an herbalist who informed me that many fake products are on the market. I have noted the current brand that I know works. This nutraceutical has been used for centuries. I personally have used it for over three decades. It also can be used as a muscle relaxer.

If you sleep on a side, keep a pillow between your legs to minimize knee pain and eliminate the possibility of causing back pain. If you are experiencing digestion problems, try sleeping on the left side. You would sleep on the right side if you do a liver cleanse. Most health advisors recommend not sleeping on your stomach.

If the weight of the blankets hurts, prop up the blankets on both the left and right sides of where you sleep. This is a common problem, according to one nurse. It is one that I currently experience. I prop my blankets up with some foam knee pads. Even books can be used. If I don't have a free space for my feet, the weight of the blankets will result in various foot pain issues.

If your neck is in pain, try getting a pillow that fits under your neck and does not tilt your head upwards when lying on your back. It took many years and untold pillow purchases before I figured this one out. Your pillow goal is to fit the area under your neck that will allow your head to maintain a natural position where the head tilts back and not upwards. If your head is forced to tilt upwards, it will distort your cervical neck and result in pain. Ultimately, it was the smallest MyPillow for women that I found helpful.

Nutrients are dosage dependent. You should be aware that the dosage required may vary with individuals regarding nutraceutical solutions for health issues. The dosage that works on a particular individual might not work on another. Therefore, some individual experimentation may be required to determine the most effective dosage for that person. Some people require a higher or lower dose based on their food and other nutrient intake. For example, my body needs about 400 mg of magnesium daily.

In contrast, my wife cannot tolerate additional magnesium because she consumes a lot of salads daily. Please only give up on a particular nutrient once you've tested it for 90 days. Your body may also need some front-loading of a nutrient. I'm sorry, but DIY health care sometimes requires that you experiment on yourself.

Some other sleep strategies I use include:

- Sleep in a dark room
- Use a sleep mask if any light is present
- Sleep in a cool room in the mid-upper 60s
- Use only enough blankets to stay warm

 God And Cancer: A Self-Care Perspective

- The weight of the blankets can help you sleep
- The weight of the blankets might prevent sleep

There are many sleep articles and videos online to help educate you.

You will need to focus and prioritize sleep so your body can rest and repair itself.

CHAPTER NINETEEN
Microbiome & Cancer

There is a growing understanding of our gut's microbiome. Some alternative health and medical professionals now believe that all disease begins inside our gut's microbiome and the diversity of its microbiota. This is the place where all food is digested. Some practitioners call the microbiome our body's second brain. Curiously, the brain has its own microbiome.

So what's going on? The microbiome communicates to our brain with instructions. Likewise, the brain communicates back to our microbiome instructions. If your microbiome is healthy and diverse, your body overall should be healthy. The reverse is also true. At least one neurologist has now tied brain disorders like ALS, Alzheimer's, Parkinson's, and other dementia disorders to an unhealthy microbiome. Likewise, cancer is also being tied to an unhealthy microbiome.

An Unhealthy Microbiome May Cause Cancer!

Our SAD (standard American diet) Western diet is now responsible for many of the severe diseases we are confronted with nowadays. I would be amiss if I didn't alert you to this as a possible cause of cancer. However, fixing your microbiome might also be a source of cure for the cancer you are experiencing.

Item 10 on page 56 in my short book[1] Healing Self-Care Primer recommends consuming a probiotic daily to help build up a more diverse microbiome. For the last two years, I have consumed a probiotic from BlueBiology[2] to build up the microbiota in my gut. However, recently, I decided to mix another brand[3] to increase the microbiome's diversity. What I like about both brands is I do not have to refrigerate them.

If you are currently sick, I would have to believe your gut's microbiome is unbalanced. In the worst situation, harmful bacteria can overwhelm good bacteria, and it could be life-threatening. If you've recently taken an antibiotic, one doctor claims it could take 6-12 months to rebuild a healthy microbiome. In any case, if you have taken treatment with antibiotics, it should be followed up by taking probiotics or consuming probiotic foods like sauerkraut, kimchi, or other probiotic-rich foods.

Your food intake can feed the body's favorable or harmful bacteria in your microbiome. If you have any doubts about the health of your microbiome, you should study this subject further. That would also pertain to any digestive issues you are experiencing.

The list of foods presented in the prior chapter on "Food & Cancer" will help you promote good microbiota diversity.

Doctors now use fecal[4] transfers from healthy people to rebuild the microbiota of people with dysbiosis[5] in their gut. Dysbiosis is a lack of balance between good and bad bacteria and plays a role in various infections and disorders, such as Clostridioides difficile infection (CFI or C. Diff), inflammatory bowel disease (IBD), cancer, periodontitis, and obesity. C. Diff[6] infections can become life-threatening as the gut microbiota becomes overwhelmed with bad bacteria. See notes for further discussion.

The use of fecal transfers has become more widely used, and in some cases, fecal pills to swallow have been created. Disgusting as it all sounds, it is saving some people from severe diseases like C. Diff.

CHAPTER TWENTY
Cancer Healing Protocols

After two decades of studying cancer, I believe that you can confidently cure your cancer using alternative health protocols. However, this assumes that you do not allow the medical industry to poison[1], burn[2], or cut[3] you by using their cancer standard of care health protocols. It is a sad fact that people with cancer often die of the medical industry's standard of care treatments rather than actually dying[4] of cancer.

DIY Healing Protocols
<u>Caveat</u>

What is the caveat in all alternative healing protocols? All of these treatments *require that you personally accept responsibility for the healing within your body.* There is no healing outside of what your body can do, and it is your body, right? So, what does this mean? You can work with an alternative cancer healing specialist who can help guide you. However, you must work on implementing the protocols or have someone in your family assist you in healing.

In contrast, we have all been trained, or more appropriately programmed, to trust the doctor for over 100 years. Remember, "the doctor knows best" is a mantra everyone alive has heard all their lives. Your family will likely pressure you to do whatever the medical doctor thinks is best.

I have a friend who recently acquired a cancer diagnosis. This person has decided to do whatever the doctor tells her to do. From a practical standpoint, that decision means the doctor controls all decision-making regarding her treatment. It places her treatments under the Medical Industry's cancer Standard of Care protocols. Medical doctors are not allowed to offer any care and advice outside of standard treatment protocols for cancer. It means the only treatment options are chemo, radiation, or surgery designed to shrink the tumor or kill cancer cells.

This means the medical doctor cannot tell you about the alternative healing protocols I'm presenting below and others you may learn from reading the book resources in the next chapter on cancer resources. Finally, it also means a certain death outcome since the medical industry's overall cure rate[5] for cancer patients may actually be as low as 2-3%[6]. Here is a quote from Dr. Leonard Coldwell's excellent book cited in the notes and as a reference guide in the next chapter.

The Only Way to Be Cured[7]

"There are no incurable diseases only incurable people. These are people who are not willing to take responsibility and take charge over their own lives. Many are not willing to accept that they have made themselves sick and therefore cannot understand that they are the only ones who have the cure within them. They usually go to their doctor and allow someone else to make all the decisions for them. Of course, they suffer a lot and finally die after having no quality of life, although they did spend a lot of money on their own 'medical suicide.' "

It's simple. Take charge of your own healing treatments, and do not let any doctor frighten you into getting poisoned, burned, or cut with their standard treatments of care. This is even more critical as Dr. Coldwell claims that 1/3rd of cancer diagnoses are false. With this caveat fully understood, let's start by examining the top three alternative cancer healing protocols I personally would use on my own body.

I personally will most likely never have a cancer diagnosis since my health strategy is to stay away from doctors and hospitals unless I have an acute health issue like a broken bone. I also have little trust in the medical industry when it comes to diagnosing or treating a chronic disease. So, from a symptom perspective, I would most likely feel lousy or off physically and first focus on detoxing the body. After detox efforts, I would use healing protocol #1. If I actually had a cancer diagnosis, I would follow all the protocols I could.

Healing Protocol #1
Oxygenate The Body

Take time to read Dr. Coldwell's book, which I've referenced in the notes and the next chapter. You'll find that oxygenating the body is the primary method he uses to cure cancer patients. Again, this assumes they have not first[8] been poisoned, burned, or cut by medical doctors. He has a documented European cancer cure rate of over 92% on over 35,000 patients, including his own family.

Oxygen kills cancer cells, a phenomenon known as the Warburg Effect. Otto Warburg[9] discovered this effect around 1930 during his experiments on cell metabolism. Cancer cells cannot survive in an oxygen-rich environment. There are many ways to increase oxygen in the body. Here is a list of ten that come to mind. I recommend the first seven low-cost methods of oxygenating the body. The last three methods should also be considered if the initial or recurring cost is not a financial obstacle.

1) Consuming Vitamin C
2) Vitamin B15 (Pangamic Acid)
3) Fresh Air Environments
4) Deep Breathing Techniques
5) 35% Hydrogen Peroxide
6) Chlorine Dioxide MMS
7) 3% Hydrogen Peroxide
8) Hyperbaric Oxygen Chamber
9) Portable Oxygen Concentrators
10) Oxygen Machine Rentals

Consuming Vitamin C

The human body naturally produces hydrogen peroxide. When Vitamin C is consumed, it increases the amount of hydrogen peroxide within the body. This then increases the oxygen in the body. Vitamin C in large quantities is known as a cancer cure. Typically, this would be in the neighborhood of 50,000 to 100,000 mg of Vitamin C, which is challenging to consume as pills. Suppose you have a healthcare practitioner willing to help you. This can be accomplished intravenously[10] with Vitamin C via an IV. For further information, see the IV protocol[11] referenced in the notes.

In a healthy body, 3-5,000 mg of Vitamin C might seem like a lot. This is especially true for a person who consumes many salads or other Vitamin C-rich foods daily. In fact, too much Vitamin C will cause loose stools or even diarrhea. However, if a body is sick or involved with a severe illness like cancer, the body can consume large amounts. Adding baking soda to regular ascorbic acid can buffer it in the stomach, making it more tolerable. There is also a buffered form of Vitamin C available to purchase.

In the past, I have built my body up to 25,000 mg a day using liquid Vitamin C. This occurred just before I contracted Covid-19 in late 2020. I published the details of my Vitamin C experiment in the book[12], *"The Doctor's Death Diagnosis."*

So, I would start consuming as much Vitamin C as my body could tolerate if I was sick with any illness. The body uses Vitamin C immediately, so the strategy would be to consume some amount at least twice an hour while I was awake. To make it as easy as possible, I would use liquid C and powdered C to make it drinkable. I could get at least 5,000 mg/hour into my body, assuming it could be used and it did not result in digestive or intestinal issues. Consuming Vitamin C is challenging, and an IV approach is a better option. If you cannot do this yourself, you will need a family member to assist.

Vitamin B15 (Pangamic Acid)[13]

B15, aka pangamate, is a nutrient derived from apricot seeds. It is a nutraceutical known to oxygenate the body. See notes for additional information. There is a purchase link[14] online to buy B15. You'll find it in the notes and on the Bonus web page referenced in the next chapter.

Fresh Air Environments

Keep the windows open inside your home to allow fresh air to circulate. Whenever possible, favor a fresh air environment. Stay out of smoke or chemically polluted areas. Try a walking version of the PACE program discussed in the prior chapter on exercise and cancer. In this version, walk as fast as possible until you are out of breath. Then stop or walk slower until you regain your breath. Repeat the process for 15 minutes. These fresh air strategies will help oxygenate your body and not cost you anything except your time.

Deep Breathing Techniques[15]

Who hasn't heard the old adage, "Take a deep breath and relax?" While deep breathing can help you relax, breathing techniques can also help oxygenate your body. See the notes for an online resource that can help you understand how mindful breathing can improve your health.

35% Hydrogen Peroxide

Madison Cavanaugh's book, "*The One Minute Cure*," thoroughly explains this process of oxygenating the body, described in the next chapter. It involves diluting food-grade hydrogen peroxide into droplets. Drops of the solution created are then added to a glass of water and drank to oxygenate the body. **Caution**: Only attempt to use 35% hydrogen peroxide after first reading all the instructions provided.

Chlorine Dioxide (CDS/MMS)

MMS (master mineral solution) is the name given to CDS (chlorine dioxide solution) by Jim Humble, who discovered its use for oxygenating the body. This process is fully explained in Jim Humble's "MMS Health Recovery Guidebook," described in the next chapter. It involves carefully mixing sodium chlorite with either hydrochloric or citric acid. Drops of the MMS solution are then added to a glass of water and drank to oxygenate the body. **Caution**: Do not attempt to use commercially available chlorine dioxide products. They would be dangerous to the body. Also, try mixing the chemicals involved only after carefully reading the mixing and dosing instructions first.

3% Hydrogen Peroxide

Hydrogen peroxide 3% solution is the standard off-the-shelve product at drug and food stores. It can be used, diluted with water, in a nebulizer to oxygenate the body. The nebulizer[16] contains a liquid chamber where you add water and some 3% hydrogen peroxide solution. Close the container and then turn the nebulizer on. You get a fine mist breathed in through the mouth or nose to oxygenate the body. This strategy can help with colds, sinus, and lung problems. **Caution**: Do not fill the container with 100% hydrogen peroxide, as it will burn. It would help if you initially filled it with 80-90% distilled or purified water and 10-20% with the hydrogen peroxide 3% solution. See how that mixture works and then gradually increase the concentration if it is comfortable to use at higher concentrations of hydrogen peroxide. Alternatively, I recommend observing and using a comprehensive nebulizer protocol like Dr. Jockers'[17]. See notes.

Hyperbaric Oxygen Chambers[18]

A hyperbaric oxygen chamber is a pressurized chamber in which the air pressure is increased to a level higher than atmospheric pressure. This allows the patient to breathe pure oxygen at higher concentrations than regular air. The process of oxygenating the body in a hyperbaric oxygen chamber involves the following three steps:

1) The patient enters the chamber, and the pressure slowly increases to the desired level, often 2 to 3 times higher than atmospheric pressure.

2) Breathing pure oxygen under increased pressure allows the lungs to absorb more oxygen, which then dissolves into the bloodstream much faster than under normal conditions.

3) The increased oxygen levels in the blood then travel to all body parts, including areas with decreased blood flow or damaged tissue. This helps promote healing and reduce inflammation.

Hyperbaric oxygen therapy is used to treat a variety of medical conditions, such as decompression sickness, non-healing wounds, carbon monoxide poisoning, and certain infections. By increasing the amount of oxygen delivered to the body, hyperbaric oxygen chambers can significantly improve the body's ability to repair and regenerate tissues, ultimately promoting healing and recovery.

In the past, these machines were expensive and limited to use at hospitals and other health institutions. However, assuming you are financially capable, these machines are now available for personal use. See notes.

Portable Oxygen Concentrators[19]

See notes for further information on portable oxygen devices.

Oxygen Machine Rentals[20]

Portable oxygen concentrators are available to rent. See notes for further information.

Healing Protocol #2
Vitamin B17 - Eat Apricot Seeds

The protocol of simply eating apricots and other fruit seeds is probably God's design for healing our bodies from cancer and other diseases. Listen to what HE says in Genesis 1:29.

And God said, "See, I have given you every herb that yields seed which is on the face of all the earth, and every tree whose fruit yields seed; to you it shall be for food."

So, what is the magic ingredient in apricot and other fruit seeds? It is Vitamin B17, which is known as Laetrile in its synthetic (drug) version. Yes, you'll find B17 in all fruit seeds. The exception, in the United States, is citrus foods. However, they are reported to still have B17 in oranges, grapefruits, and other citrus foods[21] in Africa. Our tinkering by food companies has taken B17 out of citrus foods in the U.S.

The highest concentration of B17 is found in apricot seeds. If you eat an apricot, open the hard shell encasing the seed. Inside, you will find a tender and tasty seed. The same thing is true with peaches. Apricot seeds are available to purchase in bulk[22] for eating. I have personally eaten them on and off for the last twenty years.

Apple seeds also contain B17, so you should eat the entire core when you eat an apple. Take time to crunch open the apple seeds so you can benefit from the B17. Otherwise, they'll pass through your digestive system.

There is a protocol for eating apricot seeds. Overeating too fast can make you sick. So, there are time limits to consuming apricot seeds that should be observed. Fruit seeds (B17) contain a safe form of cyanide that only attacks cancer or other unhealthy cells. The medical industry has hidden this simple cancer cure for decades. They have accomplished this by frightening people, claiming apricot seeds will kill you with cyanide poisoning. However, I've eaten them for twenty years without ill effects.

Does it really make sense that God would create fruits and tell us to eat them if the fruit and their seeds would kill us? People like the Hunza[23] live very long lives, and apricots and their seeds are a staple within their diets year-round. Cancer is non-existent in these people who live in the mountains of Northern Pakistan. You can find more information about B17 and apricot seeds on the Bonus webpage referenced in the next chapter. So, what do I know about eating apricot seeds to cure or prevent cancer?

B17 Protocol Notes

1. Apricot seeds are easy to purchase in bulk.
2. Apricot seeds are easy to eat.
3. Apricot seeds have a high concentration of B17.
4. B17 kills cancer by using a safe form of cyanide.
5. B17 kills cancer by targeting unhealthy cells with cyanide.
6. The B17 form of cyanide does not affect healthy cells.
7. Additional information is at www.1cure4cancer.com.
8. Additional information is at www.cancure.com.
9. Build your tolerance up to 20-30 seeds per day.
10. Do not exceed 7 seeds per hour or 30 per day.
11. 7-10 apricot seeds per day is a cancer prevention

strategy.

12. One seed per 10 pounds of body weight/day is safe.

13. Additional Protocols are in Dr. G. Edward Griffin's book[24].

14. Most fruit seeds contain B17. Cherries, peaches, etc.

15. B17, as Laetrile[25], is available in pill or injectable form.

16. B17 is available in 100 and 500 mg tablets.

17. B17 pills can be taken rectally if not tolerated in the stomach.

18. Both pills and seeds can be ground up and put into larger gelatin capsules rectally.

19. A complete B17 Protocol[26] Document can be found on the Bonus web page referenced in the next chapter.

20. I usually eat five apricot seeds at a time. They have a slightly bitter cherry taste and can numb the tongue, but this only lasts a few minutes.

Healing Protocol #3
The Budwig Diet

The Budwig Diet was developed in Europe in 1951 by German scientist and doctor Johanna Budwig. Shortly after hydrogenated oils became widespread, many people started suffering from various metabolic diseases like cancer[27]. Dr. Budwig took on dying patients, often with only hours or days left, and fed them flaxseed[28] oil and organic 1-2% cottage cheese.

This combination healed people by feeding electrons to the body where repairs were needed. The electrons come from the flaxseed oil, but it is fat soluble. Mixing the oil with organic cottage cheese changed it to a water-soluble solution, which the body can absorb more easily. She used this concoction to heal people for over four decades. Still, she was never able to convince science that hydrogenated oils were responsible for cancers and other health issues. Budwig believed this combination of ingredients also has the effect of oxygenating the body.

A six-time Nobel award-nominated doctor says this essential nutrient combination prevents and helps the body cure cancer! Report by Robert Willner, M.D., Ph.D.

See Willner's full report on Dr. Johanna Budwig's Diet.[29] Dr. Dan C. Roehm, M.D. FACP (Oncologist and former Cardiologist) claims that the Budwig Diet is "the most successful anti-cancer diet in the world." See notes, Willner's report for further discussion, and his optional recipes to enhance taste. So, what do I know about Dr.

Johanna Budwig's diet?

Budwig Diet Protocol Notes

1. Mix 1 cup of organic 1-2% cottage cheese with 3 tablespoons of organic liquid flaxseed oil. Eat daily.
2. Other recipes for the Budwig Diet are in the Willner report.
3. Obtain flaxseed oil from refrigerated sections only.
4. Fruit can be mixed in to make it more palatable.
5. Oxygenates the body by supplying abundant free electrons from the flaxseed oil.
6. Flaxseed oil is often referred to as linseed oil. Both come from the same plant but may contain differences, and linseed oil is primarily a commercial product.
7. Use flaxseed oil whenever doubt exists about linseed.
8. The cottage cheese makes the flaxseed oil water soluble, so the body absorbs free electrons more easily.
9. Developed in Europe by Dr. Johanna Budwig and used for over four decades as a diet cure for degenerative metabolic diseases like cancer.
10. Avoid processed foods. Many contain hydrogenated oils, which Dr. Budwig claims is the cause of the diseases.

11. As mentioned earlier, avoid seed oils high in linoleic acid. While flaxseed is similar, cottage cheese neutralizes the adverse effects.

12. Avoid lunch meats with nitric acids, which affect the body similarly to hydrogenated oils.

13. See the chapter on foods and cancer for what to eat or avoid.

14. Family help may be required for using the Budwig Diet.

15. Starve cancer cells by avoiding all sugar products.

16. Use pH strips to monitor the body's pH levels. Cancer patients are typically acidic, while healthy people are slightly alkaline. Eating greens can help restore the body to an alkaline state.

17. Cancer cannot survive in an oxygen-rich or alkaline body.

Healing Protocol #4
Molecular Hydrogen H2[30]

Molecular hydrogen H2 therapy is as simple as dropping an effervescent tablet into a glass of water. Hydrogen gas is formed in this process. As soon as the pill is dissolved, the water is drunk. Hydrogen is a powerful healer of the body. See the chapter on water & healing for further discussion, along with the article in the notes discussing 15 ways H2 can heal the body.

Healing Protocol #5
Enzyme Therapy

Adding pancreatic enzymes to the diet can enhance healing. If you use them before a meal, they will assist in the digestion of the food. Using them between meals can help destroy cancer by destroying the outer layer or casing of the cancer cells. While the enzymes attack unhealthy cells, they do not affect healthy cells. Here is an example of the two enzymes[31] I use.

Healing Protocol #6
Heat Therapy

Applying heat directly to the body near a tumor can kill the cancer. This can be accomplished with a microwave or other heating pad, or it can also be achieved using low-cost halogen utility lights. This is a DIY use of low-tech devices to heat a localized body area. You can contrast this therapy with the next one, which most likely requires an outpatient visit to a clinic or hospital.

God And Cancer: A Self-Care Perspective

Healing Protocol #7
Hyperthermia Therapy

Hyperthermia therapy is a medical treatment that uses heat to treat health conditions. It can be done by raising the temperature of a tumor or a nearby tumor or exposing the entire body to higher temperatures. This therapy can help target cancer cells and weaken or kill them. Cancer cells are more sensitive to high heat than normal healthy cells.

Hyperthermia therapy stimulates the immune system, improves blood flow, and enhances nutrient delivery to the affected area. This improves the effectiveness of other alternative cancer protocols and helps alleviate symptoms. The therapy also speeds up recovery for conditions such as infections, chronic pain, and muscle injuries.

Of course, machines are also used to increase body temperature. If you can afford professional help, visiting a medical facility as an outpatient client may be necessary.

Healing Protocol #8
Strengthen Collagen Fibers

You can strengthen the body's collagen fibers by using large doses of L-lysine[32] (10,000 mg) and a similar Vitamin C dose. This combination will help prevent cancer from spreading or metastasizing. You can also use a collagen[33] product like the one I use, which can be added to coffee in the morning to get it down. See notes.

Healing Protocol #9
Massage Therapy

Regular full-body massage can help keep the body's lymphatic system functioning. Alternatively, you can also get a lymph system massage at some locations. I am currently getting two 90-minute massages a month. This can be expensive, but family members can pitch in to do the massage or offset the cost. Keeping the lymph system healthy is essential for eliminating toxins and dead body cells. Exercise also keeps the lymph system functioning.

The lymph system does not have pipes like the circulatory system. Instead, it is the fluid that surrounds all cells. If the body is tense and tied in knots, it may not function to eliminate waste as it was designed.

Healing Protocol #10
Staying Hydrated

Staying hydrated by drinking water is essential for the body's immune system by flushing out toxins and other waste products. How much water to drink is a controversial subject. It is half my body weight in ounces. Of course, it could be different for everyone. However, many so-called diseases of the body are simply the effects of dehydration. I have a report online[34] on this subject. See notes.

Healing Protocol #11
Liquid Vitamin A

At least one cancer protocol calls for 225,000 IUs of Vitamin A daily. A liquid form[35] of Vitamin A is needed to accomplish this intake. Vitamin A can also accumulate in the liver, so caution is required. See notes.

Healing Protocol #12
Colon Cleansing

Regular colon cleansing can enhance healing. An estimated 7-21 pounds of human waste can attach itself to the walls of the large colon, and disease can breed within the waste. Cleansing the colon eliminates this waste and disease breeding; a clean colon improves the liver's ability to remove toxins. Some protocols recommend coffee animas up to 4 a day. There are many colon-cleansing products available online. Find one that works for you if it is needed.

Healing Protocol #13
Food Therapy

There is little doubt that the foods we consume can create cancer or kill cancer. The problem most of us will confront is the strong pull of our current dietary habits and the need to force more change into our lives if we expect to survive cancer. Review the chapter on Food & Cancer, and decide to eat cancer-fighting foods, even if this requires changing your taste buds, eating habits, and daily schedule. Read *Chapter 12, Fantastic Foods & Super Supplement*, in Ty Bollinger's book, *CANCER - Step Outside The Box*, for further study.

Healing Protocol #14
Nutraceutical Therapy

Dozens of nutraceuticals can assist the body in killing

cancer cells and healing efforts. I've mentioned only a few. Ty Bollinger's cancer book lists some important ones. However, a more comprehensive list is in Dr. Kevin Conners' book, "***STOP FIGHTING CANCER and Start Treating the Cause,***" referenced in the next chapter on resources. Read Conners' *Chapter 5: Nutraceuticals: 'Natural Chemotherapy'* for a comprehensive list and further study.

Healing Protocol #15
Rife Micro Current Therapy

Dr. Royal Raymond Rife was an American inventor, researcher, and scientist who developed the Rife micro-current frequency machine in the early 20th century. He believed specific frequencies could target and destroy harmful pathogens such as bacteria, viruses, and cancer cells.

The Rife machine emits electromagnetic frequencies that are believed to resonate with the unique frequencies of these pathogens, causing them to disintegrate. This process is known as frequency therapy or bio-resonance therapy.

This alternative electro-healing technology is coming of age. However, it is not accepted by allopathic medicine and is not regulatory approved for treating disease.

However, there are now decades of development and experience with micro-current frequencies in the healing of disease.

Every organ and part of the body resonates at a specific frequency, as do pathogens, bacteria, parasites, etc. This is especially true of cancer cells. These resonating frequencies are now fully understood and can be targeted successfully by micro-current devices. That means micro-current frequencies can kill cancer cells. However, you must seek treatment from a naturopath or other practitioner that uses a micro-current frequency device. Alternatively, you can buy one if you can afford it.

Dr. Keith Scott-Mumby[36] is a leading expert on small-scale, highly effective micro-current frequency devices used in healing the body. If you visit a micro-current frequency practitioner, it can cost $125-$175 for a diagnostic or treatment appointment. Purchasing a user-friendly rife device[37] currently on the market can cost from $1,500 to $5,000. I suspect renting such machines or finding used ones for sale is also possible. The frequencies[38] affecting different body organs are published online. You can watch a micro-current webinar Dr. Keith presented here[39]. He also has a lot of information on dealing with cancer on his website.

Other DIY Protocols

Other DIY healing protocols like Gerson Therapy, Protocel Therapy, Essiac Tea, Hemp, and others are discussed in the book resources shown in the next chapter. So, there is no lack of alternative healing strategies or information for you to use to cure or prevent cancer from reoccurring. Yet, to fight cancer, you have to acknowledge this is your responsibility and that you are indeed climbing a mountain. You must examine food and nutraceuticals and determine what you will use and how much alternative DIY healing expenditures you can support. From that perspective, I recommend using the first three protocols I've discussed. There is little doubt that you will need a solid reason to fight for your healing instead of just following what the doctor wants. Perhaps your reason to fight to live comes from an answer to the question: "Why am I here?"

Do you have a good reason to live?
To fight?

CHAPTER TWENTY-ONE
Cancer Resources

Recommended Reading

I have arranged these recommended books in the order that I think will help you the most in healing your cancer. The first two books I've cited should be considered mandatory reading before you follow any medical doctor's treatment regimen.

Feeling Is The Secret by Neville Goddard (1944)

This is a short spiritual book of only 28 pages in print form. It can also be found online as an eBook. You can also find it narrated in a YouTube[1] video. See note. While it is a short read and only about 45 minutes narrated online, it is a profound guide that will help you to get what you want. What do you want if you have cancer? Well, you want healing, of course. I put this book in the number one position on this list because I think it will benefit everyone with cancer. It is well-written and easy to understand. It will teach you the principle of focusing on how you feel when healed. Of course, the "feeling" principle can be applied to many areas of life where you want to succeed. This assumes you keep your focus on healing feelings and not on your cancer.

The ONLY Answer To Cancer by Dr. Leonard Coldwell

<u>BEFORE</u> you get yourself "**cut, poisoned, or burned**[2]" by allopathic medicine's cancer treatments, you should give yourself the time to read Dr. Coldwell's book. It took your body years to arrive at your cancer diagnosis. Your body will wait until you read this valuable educational resource. This Seventh Edition, published in 2011, will help you understand what you are against with a cancer diagnosis. Dr. Coldwell has treated over 35,000 cancer patients with a documented 92% cure rate. He states that "cancer is very easy to cure" as long as you don't allow your body to get cut, poisoned, or burned by traditional medical treatments.

Instinct-Based Medicine by Dr. Leonard Coldwell

In this 2008 book, Dr. Coldwell explains how, using common sense and instincts, you "can survive your illness and your doctor[3]." Focusing on stress as being responsible for 95% of all illnesses, according to a Stanford University study, Coldwell explains the body's healing process and how to eliminate disease.

Feelings Buried Alive Never Die by Karol K. Truman

A lot of stress that causes illness and diseases like cancer comes from submerged childhood traumas buried deep in our subconscious minds. They can impact our lives decades later. Humans operate during the day, with 95% of our activities on autopilot derived from whatever is deep in our subconscious. The other 5% would be conscious decisions we make daily. This means that even though you buried a childhood trauma(s) and are not consciously aware of them, they continue to impact your life until they are fully resolved. How do you know you might have buried traumas? Suppose you experience bitterness, hate, resentfulness, vengefulness, unhappiness, failure, and other negative emotions. In that case, it is a sign of possible buried traumas.

Chris Beat Cancer[4] by Chris Wark (2021, 2nd Edition)

I had the opportunity to watch a cancer healing video docuseries featuring the strategies Chris used to beat his cancer. It was a great series on curing cancer, where Chris walked you through every aspect of the healing process. Is the video series still available? You'll have to inquire at his website. Check out Chris Wark's website if you need a personal cancer coach or community feedback to guide you through a healing process. See note.

Stop Fighting CANCER and Start Treating the Cause by Dr. Kevin Conners (Third Edition, 2020)

This book is loaded with specific DIY cancer cures and is very impressive. This is a Minnesota doctor with his own clinic called the Conners Clinic. Phone consultations and visits to his clinic in Minnesota are available. Need a medical doctor practicing Integrative Cancer Therapy? This book impressed me with the doctor's familiarity and recommendations for alternative healing modalities, such as the Rife frequency machine and B17 as curative modalities. This means that this doctor knows more than 99% of other medical doctors about healing modalities for treating cancer. This book has detailed cancer advice and cures for DIY individuals. Best of all, it is backed up by a Doctor and Clinic that knows alternative healing approaches to cancer. Cures that do not involve cutting, burning, or poisoning your body.

CANCER - Step Outside The Box by Ty Bollinger (6th Edition, 2014)

This is another excellent reference guide for understanding the history of cancer treatments along with the abuse of government agencies by hiding non-toxic cancer cures. This 533-page book gives you all the details and detailed information on alternative healing cures, including foods that will help. Ty's family, like mine and others, suffered cancer deaths and no doubt experienced the abuse and ignorance of the allopathic medical industry. For those who choose to get educated during or after a cancer experience, it can be shocking to discover the kinds of detailed alternative healing information available in Ty's book.

The One-Minute CURE - The Secret to Healing Virtually All Diseases by Madison Cavanaugh (2008)

This 114-page book is your recipe for using 35% food-grade hydrogen peroxide to oxygenate your body. The process involves diluting 35% hydrogen peroxide and then using drops in eight ounces of water several times a day to bring oxygen into play within your body for healing any disease. Everything you need to know is inside this book. Only attempt to use 35% hydrogen peroxide after reading through the instructions. Without the proper dilution, it is highly toxic and can burn your skin.

Hydrogen Peroxide - Medical Miracle H2O2 by William Campbell Douglass II, MD (2003)

This book discusses various medical uses of hydrogen peroxide, including using 3% H2O2 solutions on gums and sanitizing toothbrushes.

MMS Health Recovery Guidebook - Revised Edition by Jim Humble with Cari Lloyd (2019)

I mentioned earlier the idea of using chlorine dioxide to heal your cancer. This is referred to as CDS, which adds hydrochloric acid to sodium chlorite. The entire process is simple and easy to accomplish, resulting in what is referred to as MMS or Master Mineral Solution. Once available, it is used similarly to the hydrogen peroxide drops in the One-Minute Cure book.

Jim Humble was sent home to die with multiple tumors after the medical system did all it could. He went into treatment with a few tumors. After the medical system worked on him, he was sent home to die with over 70 tumors. Jim noticed chlorine dioxide was used commercially to oxygenate water treatment plants to kill pathogens. He eventually healed himself using the same concept.

This is a recipe book on using CDS/MMS to heal your body from cancer and other diseases. I just finished another 35 hours of a docuseries called "Cancer Secrets." It was highly promoted as a cancer cure and method of oxygenating the body. Please do not attempt to mix the chemicals without first reading the entire book and its recipes and processes. You can also find a YouTube video[5] by Dr. Andreas Kalcker that illustrates the CDS mixing process. MMS is the name given to the final CDS solution by Jim Humble.

Unfortunately, the Medical Industry is in full attack mode against using MMS for healing. Of course, they do not want you to use any low-cost cure for healing disease. Treating disease is a big business, especially treating cancer. Get the book, watch the doctor's video online, and make your own decision. It is a recognized fact that Jim Humble healed himself after being sent home by the medical establishment to die of cancer.

Dissolving Illusions - Disease, Vaccines, and the Forgotten History by Suzanne Humphries, MD and Roman Bystrianyk (2015)

This is a 504-page historical review of the history of vaccines and the harm they have caused around the world. The historical evidence presented will leave little doubt in a person's mind that vaccines are harmful. Instead of immediately getting this book, take some time to view the information at the book's website, https://dissolvingillusions.com/. You will find some graphics that reveal the truth about measles and other popular vaccines promoted by the Medical Industry and Big Pharma.

If the hidden alternative cancer cure information didn't shock you, this hidden vaccine information the Medical Industry hides will shock you.

If you have a severe illness, disease, or cancer, do not subject yourself to vaccinations of any type.

All vaccines contain an adjuvant to accelerate the creation of antibodies. This adjuvant is usually aluminum or mercury, which are toxic to the body, especially the brain.

Annual flu shots are unproven to help your health and contain ingredients toxic to your brain. Therefore, if you insist on getting yearly flu shots, you are subjecting your body and brain to poisonous metals and, at some point, may be headed to early dementia or Alzheimer's.

Given the current childhood vaccine schedule and the adjuvant toxic metals they contain, why shouldn't Autism rates among children be at excessive levels in 2024. Cohort studies of vaccinated and unvaccinated children prove that vaccines are harming children. If you want the historical truth about vaccines, get this book. It is written by a medical doctor and a historical researcher. The book contains quotes from medical doctors from over the last century.

The Lost Book of Herbal Remedies - The Healing Power of Plant Medicine by Nicole Apelian, Ph.D & Claude Davis (2019)

Of all the books I have looked forward to, I was very excited to get my hands on this one. Like a lot of alternative authors, Nicole had to fight for her own healing after being diagnosed with MS (Multiple Sclerosis). I recall one interview where she indicated she was in a wheelchair. Nicole literally had to heal herself of this autoimmune disease and get out of the wheelchair. She did it with herbs.

There is a section listing all the herbs for cancer prevention and treatment. It lists the following herbs: balsam fir, bilberry, birch, bleeding heart, blue and black elderberry, cabbage, calendula, cleavers, comfrey, cranberry, dandelion, devil's club, flax, greater burdock, hardy kiwi, honey locust, leeks, lemon balm, lion's mane, mayapple, milk thistle, oregano, Oregon grape, purslane, reishi, rosemary, self-heal, Turkey tail, white mustard, and wormwood.

The book also has two other cancer lists: one for dealing with skin cancer and the other for tumors. You might recognize some of these herbs. The authors thoroughly explain them in their book. If you are as curious about herbs as I am, this is an excellent addition to your health library.

Author's Online Bonus Gift
DIY Cancer Resource Page

I have created an online healing resource to supplement this book with additional cancer resources and DIY self-care healing information as a bonus gift. As I find significant DIY cancer-fighting resources, I will add them to this online resource page. This author bonus resource page is private and can be found online at - http://www.godandcancer.org/resources.html.

This web resource is a bonus gift for the purchasers of this book. Please enter the above web address into your browser and then bookmark the page when it appears. Yes, you can share the link with family and friends. On this book's online bonus cancer resource page, you will find other significant DIY resources for your cancer studies.

One of those resources is G. Edward Griffin's explanation of the B17 fruit seed cure. Eating apricot seeds, rich in Vitamin B17, is one of my favorite cures for cancer. Eating fruit seeds like apples, apricots, and peach seeds can help avoid or heal cancer. When you eat an apple, crunch the seeds so the B17 nutrients will enter your system. If you consume apricot seeds, follow the protocol in the prior chapter. Too many apricot seeds can make you sick. You'll find a link on my Bonus page to purchase bulk apricot seeds and other DIY products for healing cancer.

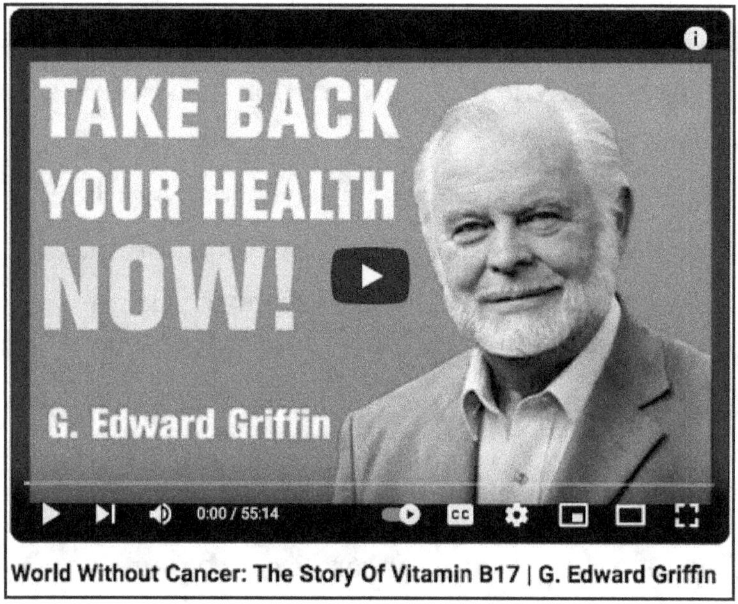

World Without Cancer: The Story Of Vitamin B17 | G. Edward Griffin

What Would Ed Do?

What if I had cancer? You will find the complete answer to this question on my health blog "What would Ed do?" It's on my author's website at http://www.edwardgpalmer.com/blog2.html.

I would heavily emphasize using the first three protocols disclosed in the prior chapter. These protocols are 1) Oxygen Therapy, 2) B17 Apricot seed therapy, and 3) Dr. Budwig's flaxseed oil and cottage cheese therapy. See my blog online for a complete discussion of why I would focus on these three cures.

Prayer

I pray that everyone who reads this book will find hope and a cure for their cancer. May God greatly bless you, heal your body, and give you a long life. *Edward*

Notes

Introduction

1. You'll find "Healing Self-Care: A DIY Primer" at http://www.healingselfcareprimer.com. This book teaches how to create a DIY self-care program to help you avoid doctors and hospitals by taking charge of your health.
2. You'll find "God And Healing" at http://www.godandhealing.org. Five book versions are available, including a $2.99 ePub and Kindle edition.
3. DIY is an abbreviation for Do-It-Yourself
4. You'll find "The Doctor's Death Diagnosis" at http://www.thedoctorsdeathdiagnosis.com. Five book versions are available, including a $2.99 ePub and Kindle edition.
5. You find "Healing Self-Care Primer" online at http://www.healingselfcareprimer.com. This book is also free from the author as a PDF download for everyone who signs up for his health and healing newsletter at his author's website at http://www.edwardgpalmer.com.
6. Jacqueline Lee Bowers,1946 -2003. We had a 43-year love story and were married for 39 years before she died. For further information, see my Eulogy at http://www.mplsvocational.com/about/dedicated-to-jackie.html. The original text used my wife's actual name, "Jackie." In this cancer update, I used the phrase "my first wife" or "my wife" in place of her actual name to take some of my emotion out of this writing.
7. This non-public website page is a bonus gift for purchasers of this book. See the Chapter on Cancer Resources for the web address to use in a browser.

The Understanding Heart

1. See the book website at http://www.godand-jesus.org for further details.

2. Virtually all Bible translations have this similar translation: Jesus stated he was a man who heard from God.

3. If you don't believe unrighteousness exists within the Christian community, visit http://www.james417.org and study Matthew 7:21-23. It is a sad fact, and the reason it is discussed here deals with how our beliefs can affect our healing. For further reading, study Matthew 13:15 and what Jesus says about our faith and healing.

4. See http://www.godand-jesus.org for a complete discussion and the other author resources listed in the back.

5. See chapter one in my book "God And Jesus: The Identity Crisis" for a more detailed discussion of our FIRST Love.

6. This discussion is about righteousness. However, there is a nagging scripture that haunts me concerning Trinity believers. When Christ returns, he takes vengeance on those who do not know his God. You'll find this teaching in 2 Thessalonians 1:8. It disturbs my soul, as many Trinity believers do not know the God whom Jesus knew.

The Stress Solution

1. I believe this rest for our souls is found only in God's love. This means rest is in the FATHER.

2. See James 4:8 for further study. Yes, if you move towards God, HE will move towards you.

3. See Proverbs 3:5.

The Appointed Time, Part 3

1. An expanded list of 66 Bible Healing Verses can be downloaded at this link - https://www.biblestudytools.com/topical-verses/healing-bible-verses/ - Note: I found several Scripture citations in this list that were in error, but the verses themselves were correct if you can find the proper location in Scriptures.

2. Unless otherwise identified by a 3-4 letter Bible identifier.

3. I have substituted God's pronoun "HE." The Bible reads "I," and may

refer to God's Angel sent to guide the Israelites. The Bible reads "I," which may refer to God's Angel sent to guide the Israelites. However, healing and the fulfillment of our days _only_ come from God, even if HE directed an angel or even Jesus Christ to make it happen for us.

4. The bracketed words are mine for clarification. Indeed, God heals us by the stripes of Jesus, who was wounded for our sins.

5. Jesus makes it clear in the Scriptures that he was given power by God and that he was delegating power to his apostles [and other believers who have not seen him].

6. The Catholic NAB Bible correctly shows that God's Spiritual power was exercised by Jesus. Therefore, God was _with_ Jesus.

7. A real believer will use the name of Jesus to create healing. So, command your healing in Jesus's name as you pray to God.

8. I replaced the word "Lord" with "Jesus". This is my perspective since Jesus taught us to pray to God in his name, and the Bible clearly teaches that healing comes from God.

9. The word "Lord" is shown in small caps since I believe it is correct that healing comes from God, even if it comes through the hands of Jesus or another person. We pray to God in Jesus' name, which is the principle I've used to interpret this verse.

10. See my book "Healing Self-Care Primer" at http:// www.healingselfcareprimer.com

11. See Genesis 6:3

12. See the Nag Hammadi library and other books that explain the Gnostic Gospel of Philip.

13. Ephesians 6:12: "For we do not wrestle against flesh and blood, but against principalities, against powers, against the rulers of the darkness of this age, against spiritual hosts of wickedness in the heavenly places."

14. An individual's spiritual union with God ALMIGHTY through acceptance of Jesus' teachings. It means that the spirits of Jesus and Yahweh will dwell within and guide an individual after the union.

15. See Ephesians 6:12-18.

16. Extracting people from crashes use powered rescue tools and equipment, including the Jaws of Life. See discussion at https:// en.wikipedia.org/wiki/Vehicle_extrication

Jesus Always Healed?

1. A known theology of the AFCM churches, aka Association of Faith Church Ministries like, Kenneth Copeland, Mac Hammond, and other similar AFCM ministries.

Water & Healing

1. See the University of Washington, Seattle's - Dr. Gerald Pollack's videos on YouTube at https://www.youtube.com/watch?v=p9UC0chfXcg and at https://www.youtube.com/watch?v=i-T7tCMUDXU

2. Cancer is also referred to as the poor man's suicide because if you just ignore it, you will eventually die. Many forms of cancer are painless and not discovered until they are at stage 3 or 4, having metastasized in other parts of the body. In other words, it might seem hopeless, and maybe it's time to let go of life. People late in their 60s or older sometimes feel it's better to let go. People need something to live for to beat cancer. Water can help you fight back if you understand all of its dynamics.

3. The "Under Your Skin: The Interstitium" video explains this body organ. https://www.youtube.com/watch?v=YbG8gVQf1GI

4. This University of California Television - (1 hour 21 minutes) video explains the role of our body's fascia in movement and function. https://www.youtube.com/watch?v=raCBeQ-gXfs

5. This process is also referred to as earthing. For further explanation, see the article at https://www.healthline.com/health/grounding

6. Alternative health proponents consider an alkaline body to be healthy and resistant to disease. Likewise, they think an acidic body is friendly to disease. When my first wife was dying from pancreatic cancer, we tested our pH levels. She tested acidic at 6.0, and I tested alkaline at 7.1.

7. Stop drinking bottled water in plastic containers. Get some glass bottles to drink out of and use highly filtered water to drink. Plastic bottles can leach chemicals into the water that mimic the female estrogen hormone.

8. H2 Source 1: https://www.mercolamarket.com/product/2715/1/h2-molecular-Hydrogen-90-per-bottle-90-day-supply. H2 Source 2:

https://drkeithsown.com/collections/frontpage/products/active-h2-ultra

9. https://secure.turapur.com/journey/TURPITCH0323WEB/1?promocode=WPITZC00&pagenumber=2&organization-abbreviation=NMG

10. The Turapur filter is a countertop pitcher with a changeable internal filter or one connected to the kitchen sink. I use the countertop pitcher, which requires the internal filter to be changed every 50 gallons of water. I change my filter every 90 days, while the manufacturer recommends changing it every 60 days.

11. Based on my studies on molecular Hydrogen (H2) enhanced drinking water, this is my opinion.

12. Deuterium-depleted water can help heal cancer. There is an "Ultimate Guide" to this subject online and at - https://www.nourishmeorganics.com.au/blogs/the-ultimate-guides/the-ultimate-guide-to-deuterium-depletion

13. There are several places to buy deuterium-depleted water. This is one such place I found on the internet. Be sure to shop around. A case of (12) 16.9-ounce bottles is $155 at this site. The bottles only contain 10 ppm of deuterium, making them suitable for cleaning the interstitium. You'll find other exciting health and healing resources on this website. https://www.drinklitewater.com/?gad_source=2&gclid=EAIaIQobChMI07fh7Ki9hAMV7lB_AB0l3QnYEAAYASAAEgI-8fD_BwE

14. See the short video at https://www.youtube.com/watch?v=S72N0bdaEJk to learn how to create deuterium-depleted water using a simple triple-freezing process anyone can do at home.

15. It is now believed that the water in our interstitium flows like a river from cell to cell. Deuterium-depleted water entering the interstitium can flush out the toxins and cancers inside.

16. Studies on deuterium are located online at - https://www.deuteriumdepletion.org/

17. Deuterium-depleted water can help heal cancer. There is an "Ultimate Guide" to this subject online at - https://www.nourishmeorganics.com.au/blogs/the-ultimate-guides/the-ultimate-guide-to-deuterium-depletion

Cancer 101

1.   This list represents some of my personal thoughts about dealing with cancer.

2.   I have this as an eBook on my iPhone. The list is on page 43 of 327, or about 11% of the book. The exact list location may vary depending on what type of device you are using and whether you are reading from a printed version.

3.   I recommend reading Coldwell's cancer book before making any major decision concerning the treatment of your cancer by standard medical practices. This book might save your life and prevent needless suffering for you and your family. Do not be rushed into decisions by medical fears presented by doctors. It took years to get to this point. Some time to consider your options will ensure you are making the right choice for your life.

4.   This is the first question Doctor Henry Ealy, ND, BCHP, from the Energetic Health Institute asks his patients before giving alternative health advice for a severe disease. When it involves the mind, it is always a spiritual issue. Go to https://www.energetichealthinstitute.org/ for natural health resources.

5.   Being proactive means looking for solutions and taking responsibility for whatever is going on in your life. It means you are not turning your life over to medical doctors so that they can make the decisions for you. It also means you are not allowing yourself to be coerced or pressured by medical professionals.

6.   Every person needs a purpose for living. Otherwise, depression sets in, and if elderly, even to the point of giving up life.

7.   Allopathic medicine seeks to treat symptoms. The focus should be on the body's health, not the disease. According to one naturopathic doctor, the disease will disappear when the body is significantly improved.

8.   This involves your mind and its ability to heal the body and explains why placebos work just as well as most pharmaceutical drugs. The mind can heal the body!

9.   See Dr. Leonard Coldwell's list and excerpts.

10. Standard medical practices for cancer seek to shrink tumors. However, in the process, they kill other cells in the body. Cutting out

a tumor or even a biopsy on one can result in spreading the cancer. The body often encapsulates a tumor to protect itself. Usually, small tumors won't grow further. Beware, the medical industry promotes fear to force you into taking fast action. Take your time to consider a course of healing action. Do not let fear dictate action.

11. See the discussion on how I would increase oxygen in my body.

12. Vegetable oils like corn, canola, etc., contain linoleic acid (Omega 6), and due to the extent it is present in our modern diets, it is a significant cause of inflammation. This inflammation leads to cancers and other diseases.

13. The use of sugar is pervasive in most foods and is often difficult to avoid altogether.

14. Plastic leaches are endocrine-disrupting chemicals like BPAs that mimic estrogen hormones. As a result, it can harm the body's natural functions. This is why avoiding plastic is best for food and water consumption, cooking, and storage. Instead, make the switch back to glass bottles and containers.

15. Our body is also a spiritual being. Many illnesses have a spiritual component. Consider carefully the prior writings about God.

16. Many cancer involves past traumas experienced as a child. Trauma is known as a cause of cancer, often resulting in a diagnosis decades after the original event. The subconscious mind can harbor negative thoughts resulting from past traumas.

17. Our lives are surrounded by toxic chemicals. It would help if you examined what soaps, cleaning agents, and other chemicals containing harmful materials are being used around you. Mold in the walls or other home parts is also an environmental issue that can affect your health.

18. Amalgam dental fillings contain mercury and are known to be toxic to the body. They should be removed and replaced with composite fillings.

19. The body may have a variety of toxic metals from vaccines, dental work, and environmental influences that cause health issues.

20. In Dr. Leonard Coldwell's book The Only Answer To Cancer, he reports that stress is the number one cause of 90% of all cancers and diseases. Therefore, your emotional or stress detox must focus on the areas stressing you out. Many stressors are past traumas buried deep

into our subconscious minds. If you have buried traumas, you may need significant mental health therapy to get rid of them. Remember that some stress is present daily and necessary for a healthy body.

21. Resolving buried unresolved childhood trauma or traumas to improve health typically involves a combination of therapeutic approaches and self-care strategies. Here is a general process that may be used:

1) **Therapy:** Seeking help from a therapist or counselor trained in trauma-informed care is crucial. Therapists may use various approaches such as cognitive-behavioral therapy (CBT), dialectical behavior therapy (DBT), EMDR (Eye Movement Desensitization and Reprocessing), somatic experiencing, or trauma-focused therapy to address the underlying issues stemming from childhood trauma.

2) **Explore the Trauma:** Through therapy, individuals can explore and identify the root causes of their trauma. This may involve revisiting past experiences, understanding how the trauma has impacted their beliefs and behaviors, and processing the associated emotions.

3) **Develop Coping Strategies:** Therapists can help individuals develop healthy coping strategies to manage emotions, triggers, and stress responses. This may include relaxation techniques, mindfulness practices, establishing healthy boundaries, and cultivating self-compassion.

4) **Healing through Expression:** Encouraging the expression of trauma-related emotions and experiences is essential in the healing process. This may involve journaling, creative outlets, or supporting groups where individuals can share their stories in a safe space.

5) **Address Physical Health:** Trauma can manifest in physical symptoms and conditions. Addressing these through medical care, regular exercise, healthy nutrition, and adequate sleep is essential. Integrating practices such as yoga, meditation, and massage can also help release stored tension in the body.

6) **Build A Support Network:** Connecting with supportive friends, family members, or community resources can benefit the healing journey. A robust support system can provide a sense of belonging, validation, and encouragement.

7) **Self-Compassion and Self-Care:** Practicing self-compassion and self-care are essential for recovering from trauma. This includes

setting boundaries, prioritizing personal needs, engaging in enjoyable activities, and treating oneself with kindness and patience. It's important to note that the process of healing from childhood trauma is unique to each individual, and it may take time and patience. Seeking professional guidance and support is critical to navigating this journey towards improved health and well-being. Be aware that this process may involve long-term mental health therapy.

Remember the spiritual solution in Chapter 4 - **The Stress Solution**.

Finally, Dr. Coldwell's solution is to just let the past trauma go and move on with your life instead of spending years in psychotherapy.

22. Intermittent and time-restricted fasting will produce ketones. This is considered better overall for brain health since your brain works better with glucose.
23. If God didn't make it, don't eat it, which is the main advice concerning what constitutes a whole food item.
24. See Dr. Brownstein's Vitamin D protocol. I think it is in his book at this URL - https://www.drbrownstein.com/shop/p/a-holistic-approach-to-viruses
25. Hyperthermia involves increasing the body temperature around cancer. It can cause cancer cells to die. While the medical industry has several methods to do this safely, using a hot pad or a shop halogen lamp to increase the temperature around cancer can be a low-cost DIY method of killing cancer cells.
26. The majority of this paragraph is the exact thoughts of Dr. Leonard Coldwell, as expressed in his book "The ONLY Answer To Cancer." They are included here because the author believes it is essential for his opinions on cancer treatment to be fully understood before undergoing allopathic standard-of-care cancer treatments.

Nutrition & Cancer

1. https://capsuledepot.com/ is one example. Be sure to shop around for the best prices.
2. See this website for anal cleaning advice - https://www.healthline.com/health/how-to-clean-inside-your-bum#how-

to-wipe

3. The collagen product my wife and I use is at - https://
    www.nativepath.com/

4. According to a report by Grand View Research, the global cancer
    therapeutics market size was valued at $144.6 billion in 2020 and is
    expected to reach $274.6 billion by 2028.

5. An industry insider might say: "There are instances where efforts
    have been made to regulate or restrict certain forms of alternative
    medical information. This is often done in the interest of protecting
    public health and safety, as alternative approaches may lack scientific
    evidence or have potential risks associated with them." I would say
    that Big Pharma and the Medical Industry want to limit all forms of
    natural healing strategies.

6. And God said, "See, I have given you every herb that yields seed
    which is on face of all the earth, and every tree whose fruit yields
    seed; to you it shall be for food." Genesis 1:29

7. You can find a link to where to purchase apricot seeds in bulk on my
    cancer bonus web page at http://www.godandcancer.org/
    resources.html, and other cancer-fighting information.

8. There are many sources of liquid Vitamin C online. Choose a
    liposomal form to get a larger volume inside your body.

9. Those three-letter government agencies like the CDC, FDA, FTC, and
    others assist Big Pharma, the Medical Industry, and the Food
    Industry in making it difficult to disseminate alternative healing and
    nutritional information.

10. See my health blogs at http://www.edwardgpalmer.com for further
    healing information. See the "What Would Ed Do?" blog, which
    answers some healing questions. This is where I address feedback
    from people who search for healing information for the disease they
    have. Having already failed to find an answer, they are asking me
    what I would do if I had their disease. This is not medical advice. It is
    my perspective on a course of action I would take if I were in their
    shoes. Please read the disclaimers. I am NOT a doctor.

11. http://www.edwardgpalmer.com

12. See Genesis 6:3

13. See Jeremiah 29:11

Sugar & Cancer

1.　Dr. Frank Shallenberger's newsletter is at - https://www.secondopinionnewsletter.com/#

He has a searchable database of articles. It contains information on cancer and other health issues.

2.　See the article at https://health.clevelandclinic.org/avoid-the-hidden-dangers-of-high-fructose-corn-syrup-video for further study.

Food & Cancer

1.　This discussion of how our food choices affect cancer in our bodies is not meant to be all-encompassing. Instead, it is a general guide to help you start making healthier food choices. It is up to you to examine your current food choices and determine how to improve your health by making healthier choices.

2.　https://foodrevolution.org/

3.　There is a lot of information online about foods that can fight cancer. This is a list of 25 that I found.

4.　See article at https://www.newsmax.com/health/health-news/ultra-processed-foods-illness/2024/02/29/id/1155395/

5.　Item #3 on the list of cancer-fighting foods.

6.　*Confidential Cures*, Al Sears, 2024, p135.

Exercise & Cancer

1.　James Fixx's story is at https://en.wikipedia.org/wiki/Jim_Fixx

2.　Dr. Joseph Mercola January 08, 2024 newsletter - *"Take a Stand: The Dangers of Prolonged Sitting."*

3.　See the noted article for further details and study.

4.　You lose any benefit beyond 40-60 minutes, and over 130-140 minutes, you can end up worse than people who don't strength train.

5.　Mercola suggests that about 75 minutes of high-intensity exercise can improve health. However, beyond four hours a week, health does not improve, and the risk of heart problems increases.

6.　Mercola states that there are 2,000 steps per mile, and every additional 1,000 steps daily reduces mortality by 10% to 15%. While walking benefits plateau at 12,000 steps, they do not decrease or become counterproductive in contrast to doing too much high-intensity exercise.

7.   https://alsearsmd.com/pace-exercise-program/

8.   Although some words were changed, the following description is taken from his website.

9.   Dr. Sears has updated his PACE program as indicated in the discussion. Ensure you get his latest program notes to pursue this HIIT exercise strategy.

Teeth & Cancer

1.   The complete story is found at http://www.thedoctorsdeathdiagnosis.com.

2.   One holistic cancer specialist recommends a zirconia implant. According to https://advanceddentalartsnyc.com/everything-about-zirconia-implants/ - "Zirconia, also known as zirconium-dioxide, is a material chemically derived from zircon. It consists of Zirconium and Oxygen elements. While zirconium is a metal, due to the oxidation, Zirconia is a ceramic material. Thanks to its transitional metal status, Zirconia combines the strength of metal with the heat-resistant power of ceramic." See the website for a complete understanding of this new implant dental option.

Sleep & Cancer

1.   Boswellia is Indian Frankincense and one of the three gifts the wise men gave to the baby Jesus in the Bible. Vitacost is the brand I use, and it is relatively inexpensive. Go to - https://www.vitacost.com/vitacost-boswellia-extract-standardized

2.   https://www.vitacost.com/vitacost-synergy-mega-efa-1200-mg-omega-3-epa-dha-per-serving

3.   https://www.vitacost.com/now-borage-oil-1000-mg-60-softgels

4.   https://www.vitacost.com/vitacost-bromelain?ta=bromelain&t=bromelain

5.   https://www.vitacost.com/vitacost-gaba-gamma-aminobutyric-acid?ta=gaba&t=gaba

6.   https://www.vitacost.com/vitacost-l-theanine?ta=L-Theanine&t=l-theanine

7. https://www.vitacost.com/vitacost-melatonin-1-mg-300-capsules?ta=melatonin+1mg&t=melatonin+1mg

8. An anti-aging doctor whose clinic is in Florida, USA.

9. https://www.vitacost.com/natural-balance-happy-camper-kava-kava-root-extract?ta=kava+kava&t=kava+kava

Microbiome & Cancer

1. This is a 99-cent eBook found at http://www.healingselfcareprimer.com or free for signing up for my newsletter at http://www.edwardgpalmer.com. Wait 10 seconds for the dropdown form.

2. https://bluebiology.com/products/bluebiotics-ultimate-care

3. https://www.vitacost.com/vitacost-probiotic-15-35-15-strains

4. https://www.hopkinsmedicine.org/health/treatment-tests-and-therapies/fecal-transplant

5. See article at https://pubmed.ncbi.nlm.nih.gov/36280324/

6. https://www.c-difficile-treatment.com/ad/c-diff-colitis/?msclkid=c8d6357f122c1cd46fe15348abd944d5

Cancer Healing Protocols

1. See the chemotherapy video on my Bonus webpage, which will be disclosed in the next chapter. Chemo destroys the bone marrow in our bodies. Strangely, this process can assist in the healing of blood cancers like Lymphoma. However, in all other cancers, chemo will kill you faster than the cancer will. The chemo video on the Bonus webpage is an interview with Dr. Nicolas Gonzales, M.D., a renowned alternative doctor known for curing cancer.

2. If you allow a doctor to radiate a cancer tumor, it will also kill healthy cells and harm your immune system.

3. The body forms a shell around cancer tumors. If you allow a doctor to cut into a tumor, the cancer cells immediately spread throughout the body.

4. Before allowing any cancer treatment by the medical industry to be imposed on your body from fear, take the time to read Dr. Coldwell's "The ONLY cure for Cancer" book referenced in the next chapter. You will NEVER regret doing some homework on curing your cancer. It

took your body years to get to this cancer; your body will wait the necessary time to get educated on a healing strategy that works.

5.   The Medical Industry counts cancer as cured by their treatments if a patient survives five years. This means that if someone dies anytime after five years and one day, the industry tracks that as a cure statistic.

6.   See Dr. Coldwell's "The ONLY Cure For Cancer" book stats.

7.   This quote is found on pages 109-110 of 327 on the iPhone Kindle version of Dr. Coldwell's "The Only Cure For Cancer."

8.   You cannot expect to be rescued by an alternative healing protocol if your body has been first poisoned, burned, or cut by medical doctors. Their whole standard of care can kill healthy cells and spread cancer cells throughout the body.

9.   https://hub.jhu.edu/2021/06/04/ravenous-otto-warburg-sam-apple/

10.   You may be able to find a health care service that will do intravenous Vitamin C by searching on www.orthomolecular.org. Alternatively, try www.doctoryourself.com.

11.   You will find a Vitamin C IV Protocol at this link - http://www.doctoryourself.com/RiordanIVC.pdf.

12.   http://www.thedoctorsdeathdiagnosis.com

13.   See full explanation of B15 at https://www.apricotpower.com/blog/Vitamin-B15-Pangamic-Acid-Everything-You-Need-to-Know-Its-Benefits

14.   https://www.rawfoodandvitamins.com/

15.   https://positivepsychology.com/deep-breathing-techniques-exercises/

16.   See a portable nebulizer product at https://www.amazon.com/Portable-Nebulizer-Adjustable-Nebulization-Handheld/dp/B0CXJ8ZZGY/ref=sr_1_4?

dib=eyJ2IjoiMSJ9.lEMeRXQCceI89ENU5quSY3ElRAh9sXoKfwjB9ObS_5RvjVWFQIhbwL7ve9Mds5daDrRGVDDlO8IRzXd8TFnDzRwgW3bYdkIFfe2WsnmKKWDmZPptSfxAIyi4hfhGpUQ5M_bAFyh3gf_S8wl09r-Z2YVhWswQTAaAYTtRSTmb1vW56PS6Oe6um7e662nuOHd2asMhCxD26pwhFGfs6qliaAVhcA3BaTK_Bihi-LHS6QE.iWWKDMnbLfP7qSBbApvDQkRIApaHO3DrMOqwDvwf

Oi8&dib_tag=se&keywords=nebulizer&qid=1713385039&sr=8-4

17. https://drjockers.com/nebulizing/

18. The following website illustrates the types of hyperbaric oxygen machines available. See the website at https://www.macypanhbot.com/

19. https://www.ncoa.org/adviser/oxygen-machines/best-portable-oxygen-concentrators/

20. https://www.inogen.com/oxygen-therapy/purchase-options/

21. https://www.livestrong.com/article/250786-list-of-citrus-foods/

22. https://www.rawfoodandvitamins.com/

23. https://www.verywellhealth.com/the-hunza-valley-the-original-shangri-la-2224049

24. World Without Cancer book and video reference in the last chapter.

25. See the Bonus web page for links to purchase B17 in pill or injectable form.

26. http://godandcancer.org/files/b17_ultimate_guide.pdf

27. Many alternative doctors and health professionals believe that cancer is a metabolic disease of the body caused by malfunctioning cells.

28. https://theheartdietitian.com/linseed-vs-flaxseed/

29. http://godandcancer.org/files/Budwig_Cancer_Cure.pdf

30. See article for 15 ways H2 can heal your body at https://www.jillcarnahan.com/2018/10/14/15-science-backed-benefits-of-molecular-hydrogen-you-need-to-know-about/

31. https://www.vitacost.com/vitacost-synergy-super-daily-enzymes - and, https://www.vitacost.com/now-chewable-papaya-enzymes-360-lozenges

32. https://www.healthygoods.com/blogs/news/health-benefits-of-the-lysine-and-vitamin-c-combination

33. https://www.nativepath.com/products/original-collagen-peptides

34. http://godandcancer.org/files/Water_For_Healing.pdf

35. https://www.amazon.com/Klaire-Labs-Micellized-Vitamin-Liquid/dp/B004JP675O

36. https://alternative-doctor.com/

37. https://jwlabs.com/

38. https://www.faim.org/introduction-to-frequency-specific-microcurrent

39. https://alternative-doctor.com/micro-current-therapy-webinar-

replay/

Cancer Resources

1. https://www.youtube.com/watch?v=NqT2PzQX0Ks
2. Cut, poisoned, or burned is how Dr. Coldwell describes the ineffective methods of allopathic medicine's treatment of cancer. These methods harm you more than help you, and this book explains why.
3. The subtitle of this book is "How to survive your illness and your doctor."
4. https://www.chrisbeatcancer.com/
5. https://www.youtube.com/watch?v=3dDsjd4u7i4

Bible Translation Notes

Permissions have not been sought to quote from the following Bible translations, and the use of all copyrighted citations in this book is considered fair use under the United States copyright laws, which govern the publication of scholarly works.

A capitalization protocol has been introduced into many cited texts that make a clear distinction between God Almighty [Yahweh] and His only begotten human Son, Jesus Christ [Yashua].

Therefore, the cited text may not conform precisely to the printed Bible text used herein regarding any capitalized characters. Also, some verses are only partially presented for the sake of brevity in this book. The reader is therefore encouraged to examine all Bible citations while reading their own Holy Bible translation for a complete understanding of God's Holy Word.

1 -- (1611) The Authorized King James Version (KJV). Comment: The KJV is in the public domain in the United States and is, therefore, freely used and quoted by many people. Also, anyone can freely publish the KJV Bible.

2 -- (1982) Holy Bible, New King James Version (NKJV). Nashville, Tennessee: Thomas Nelson, Inc. Copyright © 1979, 1980, 1982. Comment: The NKJV is an update to the KJV and closely parallels the KJV text. In the author's opinion, the NKJV Bible is an excellent way to enjoy the KJV without getting entangled in comprehending its archaic and outdated English.

3 -- (1987) The Amplified Bible (AMP). La Habra, California: The Zondervan Corporation and the Lockman Foundation.

4 -- (1901) American Standard Bible (ASB) or (ASV). This Bible is in the public domain in the United States.

5 -- Berean Study Bible or The Holy Bible, Berean Standard Bible, BSB Copyright © 2016, 2020 by Bible Hub. Pittsburgh, PA 15045 USA http://www.Biblehub.com

6-- (CEB), Scripture taken from the Common English Bible®, CEB® Copyright © 2010, 2011 by Common English Bible.™ Used by permission. All rights reserved worldwide.

7 -- (CEV) Scripture quotations marked (CEV) are from the Contemporary English Version Copyright © 1991, 1992, 1995 by American Bible Society. Used by Permission.

8 -- Complete Jewish Bible (CJB), © 1998 by Messianic Jewish Publishers and Resources. Used by permission.

9 -- (CSB), Scripture quotations marked CSB have been taken from the Christian Standard Bible®, Copyright © 2017 by Holman Bible Publishers. Used by permission.

10 -- Darby Bible (DB), John Nelson. Public Domain, 1833.

11 -- (DRC1752) Douay-Rheims 1752. This Bible is in the public domain.

12 -- (EMTV) English Majority Text Version. Copyright © 2009 By Paul W. Esposito, Used by permission of the copyright holder Courtesy of Stauros Ministries.

13 -- (ENO) Book of Enoch, Richard Laurence 1883 Edition. This book is in the public domain.

14 -- (ESV) English Standard Version. Scripture quotations are from The ESV® Bible (The Holy Bible, English Standard Version®), copyright © 2001 by Crossway, a publishing ministry of Good News Publishers. Used by permission.

15 -- (1978) Good News Bible (GN). Copyright by American Bible Society. New York: Thomas Nelson Publishers. Aka "The Bible in Today's English Version;" or "Today's English Version."

16 -- (1978) Good News Bible; with Deuterocanonicals/ Apocrypha (GNBA). Copyright by American Bible Society. New York: Thomas Nelson Publishers. Aka "The Bible in Today's English Version; with Apocrypha."

17 -- (GNV) Geneva Bible 1560. This Bible is in the public domain.

18 -- (1995) God's Word (GW). Copyright by the Nations Bible Society. Bible database © 1997 by NavPress Software at www.wordsearchbible.com.

19 -- (HCSB) Holman Christian Standard Bible. Scripture quotations marked HCSB are taken from the Holman Christian Standard Bible®, Used by Permission HCSB ©1999, 2000, 2002, 2003, 2009 Holman Bible Publishers. Holman Christian

20 -- (JPS) Mamre, Mechon (2002) The Hebrew Bible in English according to the JPS 1917 Edition; HTML Version (HEB). Internet: http:www.mechon-mamre.org.

21 -- (ISV) International Standard Version. Scripture is taken from the Holy Bible: International Standard Version® Release 2.0. Copyright © 1996-2013 by the ISV Foundation. Used by permission of Davidson Press, LLC.

22 -- (JSB) Jewish Study Bible. Berlin, Adele and Brettler, March Zvi (Editors) 1985, 1999, 2004. Jewish Publication Society, Oxford, New York: Oxford University Press.

23 -- (LIV aka TLB) Scripture quotations are taken from The Living Bible, copyright © 1971 by Tyndale House Foundation. Used by permission of Tyndale House Foundation, Carol

Stream, Illinois 60188. All rights reserved.

24 -- (MACE NT) David Mace's 1729 New Testament. This Bible is in the public domain.

25 -- (MEV) Modern English Version Bible. Scripture is taken from the Modern English Version. Copyright © 2014 by Military Bible Association. Used by permission.

26 -- (MLT) 1988 Morris Literal Translation. Copyright by Ellis Enterprises, Inc., Oklahoma City, OK. See "The Bible Library" software.

27 -- (MOFF) Moffatt, James A. R. (1922, 1924, 1925, 1926, 1935, 1950, 1952 and 1954). The Bible: James Moffatt Translation (MOF). Final Edition used and Copyrighted in 1994 by Kregel Publications, Grand Rapids, Michigan.

28 -- (MSG) The Message Bible. Scripture quotations marked MSG are taken from The Message, copyright © 1993, 2002, 2018 by Eugene H. Peterson. Used by permission of NavPress. All rights reserved. Represented by Tyndale House Publishers.

29 -- (NAB) The New American Catholic Bible. Scripture texts in this work are taken from the New American Bible, revised edition © 2010, 1991, 1986, 1970 Confraternity of Christian Doctrine, Washington, D.C., and are used by permission of the copyright owner.

30 -- (NABRE) The New American Bible - Revised Edition. Scripture texts in this work are taken from the New American Bible, revised edition © 2010, 1991, 1986, 1970 Confraternity of Christian Doctrine, Washington, D.C., and are used by permission of the copyright owner.

31 -- (1970) New American Standard Bible (NASB). "Scripture quotations taken from the (NASB®) New American Standard Bible®, Copyright © 1960, 1971, 1977, 1995, 2020 by The

Lockman Foundation. Used by permission. All rights reserved. lockman.org"

32 -- (NASB77) The New American Standard Bible, 1977. "Scripture quotations taken from the (NASB®) New American Standard Bible®, Copyright © 1960, 1971, 1977, 1995, 2020 by The Lockman Foundation. Used by permission. All rights reserved. lockman.org"

33 -- (NASB1995) The New American Standard Bible, 1995. "Scripture quotations taken from the (NASB®) New American Standard Bible®, Copyright © 1960, 1971, 1977, 1995, 2020 by The Lockman Foundation. Used by permission. All rights reserved. lockman.org"

34 -- (NASB2020) The New American Standard Bible, 2020. "Scripture quotations taken from the (NASB®) New American Standard Bible®, Copyright © 1960, 1971, 1977, 1995, 2020 by The Lockman Foundation. Used by permission. All rights reserved. lockman.org"

35 -- (NCV) 1991 The Holy Bible, New Century Version. Aka, "The Everyday Bible." Dallas, Texas: Word Publishing. Comment: Excellent modern English translation.

36 -- (NET) The New English Translation. Scripture quoted by permission. Quotations designated (NET) are from the NET Bible® copyright ©1996, 2019 by Biblical Studies Press, L.L.C. https://netbible.com

37 -- (NET1) The New English Translation - First Edition. Scripture quoted by permission. Quotations designated (NET) are from the NET Bible® copyright ©1996, 2019 by Biblical Studies Press, L.L.C. https://netbible.com

38 -- (NIV) 1984 The Holy Bible, New International Version. Copyright by International Bible Society. Published by Zondervan Bible Publishers.

39 -- (NIV2011) The New International Version, 2011. Zondervan is granting permission for the latest edition of the NIV text only (currently 2011.) We are not granting permission for use of the earlier editions or versions of the NIV text. Early text may be cited due to the scholarly nature of this book.

40 -- (NJB) 1985 The New Jerusalem Bible. Copyright by Darton, Longman & Todd Ltd and Doubleday, a division of Bantam Doubleday Dell Publishing.

41-- (NLT) Scripture quotations marked (NLT) are taken from the Holy Bible, New Living Translation, copyright ©1996, 2004, 2015 by Tyndale House Foundation. Used by permission of Tyndale House Publishers, Carol Stream, Illinois 60188. All rights reserved.

42 -- (NMV) The New Messianic Version Bible. Copyright TOV Rose from 2000-2018. Citations, if used, are under the fair use doctrine for scholarly writings.

43 -- (NRSV) 1989 New Revised Standard Version. Copyright by Division of Christian Education of the National Council of Churches of Christ in the United States of America. Zondervan Publishing House.

44 -- (NRSV-CI) New Revised Standard Version, Catholic Confessional Edition. Copyright by Division of Christian Education of the National Council of Churches of Christ in the United States of America. Zondervan Publishing House.

45 -- (NRSVUE) New Revised Standard Version, 2021. Copyright by Division of Christian Education of the National Council of Churches of Christ in the United States of America. Zondervan Publishing House.

46 -- (REB) 1989 The Revised English Bible. Copyright by Oxford University Press and Cambridge University Press.

Comment: The Revised English Bible is a revision of The New English Bible.

47 -- (RSV) 1952 Revised Standard Version. Copyright by Division of Christian Education of the National Council of Churches of Christ in the United States of America. Zondervan Publishing House.

48 -- (SET) 1981 Simple English Translation, New Testament. Copyright by International Bible Translators, Inc.

49 -- (TAN) Scherman, Nosson and Zlotowitz, Meir (General Editors). (1996) The Stone Edition, Tanach. Brooklyn, New York: Mesorah Publications, Ltd.

50 -- (TEV) Today's English Version Bible. Today's English Version was first published as a full Bible in 1976 by the American Bible Society as a "common language" Bible. It provides a clear and simple modern translation. Content and copyright are believed to be the same or similar to the GB or GNT bibles.

51 -- (WEB) Noah Webster's Bible, 1833, Public Domain.

52 -- (WEY) Clarke, J. Public Domain, 1909. Weymouth's New Testament.

53 -- (WESLEY NT) John Wesley's New Testament. This Bible is in the Public Domain.

54 -- (YLT) Young, Robert. Public Domain, 1898. Young's Literal Translation.

About The Author

Edward G. Palmer has studied alternative health and healing issues for over 50 years. He considers himself a "DIY Healing Self-Care" expert and is sought after for his alternative healing and nutraceutical strategies.

He took his first comprehensive multivitamin at the age of 25 in 1971. Already in excellent health and with plenty of energy, Ed was surprised at how this multivitamin enhanced his health and vitality in a way he could not deny. That early life experience began a lifelong effort to use vitamins and other nutraceuticals, such as herbs, to enhance his health.

Ed quickly concluded that he could not bet his health on being able to eat well. Instead, Ed decided he would eat the healthiest he could but would bet his overall health and longevity on nutraceuticals.

As a child, Ed's parents taught him by their own example to care for himself and not rely on doctors for his health and healing. The biggest lesson learned early in life was that we are all personally responsible for our own health.

Author & Publisher

Author Information

Edward G. Palmer

13570 Grove Drive #361

Maple Grove MN 55311

http://www.edwardgpalmer.com

Publisher Information

JVED Publishing

13570 Grove Drive #361

Maple Grove MN 55311

http://www.jvedpublishing.org

Related Self-Care Health Books

God And Healing: A Bible Perspective

This 6 x 9" book discusses what the Bible says about Divine healing. Will God always heal as a result of prayer? It is available in Print, PDF, and $2.99 eBook editions. Details at http://www.godandhealing.org

The Doctor's Death Diagnosis

This 6 x 9" book discusses alternative healing strategies to allopathic medicine. It has a list of "100 Healing Secrets & Tips." It is based on the author's 50-year experience using alternative health strategies. It is available in softcover Print, hardcover Print, low-cost PDFs, and $2.99 eBooks. Details at http://www.thedoctorsdeathdiagnosis.com.

Healing Self-Care Primer

This 6 x 9" book teaches you "How To Create a DIY Self-Care Health & Healing Program" to help you tap into the body's healing capacity, reduce medical costs, and promote overall health. It is a short book that encourages readers to reclaim their health, freedom, and life through self-care principles and an alternative perspective on healthcare. It is available in softcover print, low-cost PDFs, and $.99 eBooks. Details are found at http://www.healingselfcareprimer.com.

Other Books & Writings

Several other books are available and several free to read writings of the author. You can find them at the publisher's website. The free writings are found towards the bottom of the publisher's home page. http://www.jvedpublishing.org.

A Real Salvation Prayer

OPENING PRAYER: *FATHER God, let everyone who utters this prayer of salvation unto YOU, with a sincere heart, immediately feel the presence of YOUR Holy Spirit and equip them with the internal strength of conviction to stand tall for YOUR righteousness at all costs and even unto their human death. Verily I say unto YOU that this is YOUR expectation of their [and my] sincere heart. Edward*

INSTRUCTIONS: Pray out loud and offer up to God ALMIGHTY outstretched arms and the following prayer, on your knees, in the privacy of your prayer closet [private room, alone], and with your sincere heart. Verily I say unto you that your soul will see eternal life in heaven upon the death of your earthly body if your heart is honest with God to the point that your behavior turns to HIS righteousness. Mark down the time, date, and place of this gift of your heart unto God, and feel free to share this moment when you committed to walking in God's ways with HIS priorities over your life.

PRAY Heavenly FATHER, the only ONE and True God. YOU, who are also the FATHER and the only ONE and True God of my brother Jesus Christ whom YOU sent down as a living human sacrifice for the sins of all the humans in this earthly realm and world, hear this prayer from my sincere heart. This prayer comes from within the bowels of my spirit soul, and I fully understand that this is a one-way decision of my committed heart.

FATHER, I believe in YOUR only human begotten Son, Jesus Christ. I believe that YOU sent Christ down to this earth and that he became the human being Jesus Christ [Yashua] in the flesh, just like the flesh I have. I believe he had bones like I do, flesh like I do, and blood like I do. I believe that his body on the cross was no different from any other human body. I acknowledge Jesus Christ is the Son of God; he is not God.

FATHER, I believe he only spoke what YOU told him to say and did what YOU told him to do. I believe that he was the final and perfect blood sacrifice for the forgiveness of the sins of humanity. FATHER, I believe that includes my sins.

LORD, I fully acknowledge that by accepting Jesus Christ as my savior and brother, I am inviting his perfect spirit into my life to share this earthly body with me. Along with his spirit, I understand that YOU will also give me YOUR Holy Spirit and that YOU also will dwell within me.

I believe that the result of my sincere acceptance of this gift of YOUR Son is the Oneness I will share with YOU and him. Christ has taught me that I might live in perfect Oneness, Peace, and Joy with YOU and him. O LORD, this is genuinely the sincere desire of my heart. I no longer want to be spiritually alone.

Therefore, I accept the precious gift of YOUR Son, Jesus Christ, and I repent of my past sins and sincerely regret every thought, action, behavior, or anything that was displeasing unto YOU. I understand that with the precious gift of YOUR Son, YOU expect me to live a righteous life for the rest of my days on this earth.

Such a life entails living up to YOUR expectations and obeying what YOU and YOUR Son taught us in Holy Scripture. LORD, I acknowledge that I cannot be perfect in and of myself. I realize that to be like Christ requires that I "practice righteousness" and avoid sin to the best of my ability. I acknowledge that to continue willfully to sin is an implicit rejection of the gift of Jesus.

I also acknowledge FATHER that there will be unintentional and unknown sins that will come in my life. I understand that YOU and Christ will cover those types of sin and serve as a guide to keep me on the narrow path to heaven.

FATHER, I acknowledge that YOUR Son is not a free pass on sins like many Christians believe. Therefore, when I realize I have sinned against YOU in any way, I promise to confess that sin immediately and to keep a short list of my missteps with YOU. I know YOU are faithful to forgive under such conditions, but I also realize that if any life is filled with such confessions, it will be a testimony of an insincere heart. I recognize YOUR instructions in Ezekiel 18 and that Jesus has not altered YOUR criteria for punishing sinners. Therefore, keep me under YOUR wings, O God, and give me a pure heart unto YOU.

Having said this, FATHER, I pray that you will dwell within me and help me be the man [or woman] you want me to be. I ask all this in the name of Jesus Christ, whom I confess with my mouth that he came in the flesh as YOUR only begotten Son. I acknowledge with my heart that YOU expect righteousness, a new life with changed behavior that glorifies YOU.

FATHER, help me to be an instrument of YOUR will even as Christ was such an instrument. Let this day be the first day of the rest of my life, and help me to put away all offensive behavior and sin, which YOU hate. I pray in the name of YOUR only begotten and beloved human Son, Jesus. **AMEN**

Record Of Prayer

Date: _______________________________________

Time:_______________________________________

Place:_______________________________________

I Told: ______________________________________

____

Salvation Prayer Scriptures

John 17:3
- Knowing the ONE true God is Eternal Life
- Knowing that God sent Jesus

John 8:40
- Jesus claimed he was a man [human male]

John 20:17
- Jesus claimed he had a God [the FATHER]
- Jesus claimed his God was also our God

Matthew 4:10
- Jesus taught us to worship only his God

Romans 10:9-13
- Confess with the mouth, Jesus
- Believe that God raised Jesus
- Believing in your heart unto God's righteousness
- Calling on the name of God, aka YAHWEH (LORD)

1 John 3:7
- If we practice righteousness, we are like Christ

John 14:23
- We can become One with Jesus and God

James 4:17
- Not doing what is right is a sin
- Defines sin regardless of education

Ezekiel 18
- God's repentance criteria in Old Testament
- Same as John the Baptist in N.T.
- Same as Jesus Christ in N.T.

Reader Notes

Reader Notes

God And Cancer: A Self-Care Perspective

Reader Notes

www.ingramcontent.com/pod-product-compliance
Lightning Source LLC
Chambersburg PA
CBHW061027250726
48659CB00015B/1053